T0231523

NEUROVISION REHABILITATION GUIDE

NEUROVISION REHABILITATION GUIDE

Amy Chang

Steven E. Ritter

Xiao Xi Yu

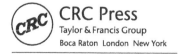

CRC Press
Taylor & Francis Group
Boca Raton London New York

CRC Press is an imprint of the
Taylor & Francis Group, an **informa** business

CRC Press
Taylor & Francis Group
6000 Broken Sound Parkway NW, Suite 300
Boca Raton, FL 33487-2742

© 2016 by Taylor & Francis Group, LLC
CRC Press is an imprint of Taylor & Francis Group, an Informa business

No claim to original U.S. Government works

Printed on acid-free paper
Version Date: 20160406

International Standard Book Number-13: 978-1-4987-6256-4 (Paperback)

This book contains information obtained from authentic and highly regarded sources. While all reasonable efforts have been made to publish reliable data and information, neither the author[s] nor the publisher can accept any legal responsibility or liability for any errors or omissions that may be made. The publishers wish to make clear that any views or opinions expressed in this book by individual editors, authors or contributors are personal to them and do not necessarily reflect the views/opinions of the publishers. The information or guidance contained in this book is intended for use by medical, scientific or health-care professionals and is provided strictly as a supplement to the medical or other professional's own judgement, their knowledge of the patient's medical history, relevant manufacturer's instructions and the appropriate best practice guidelines. Because of the rapid advances in medical science, any information or advice on dosages, procedures or diagnoses should be independently verified. The reader is strongly urged to consult the relevant national drug formulary and the drug companies' and device or material manufacturers' printed instructions, and their websites, before administering or utilizing any of the drugs, devices or materials mentioned in this book. This book does not indicate whether a particular treatment is appropriate or suitable for a particular individual. Ultimately it is the sole responsibility of the medical professional to make his or her own professional judgements, so as to advise and treat patients appropriately. The authors and publishers have also attempted to trace the copyright holders of all material reproduced in this publication and apologize to copyright holders if permission to publish in this form has not been obtained. If any copyright material has not been acknowledged please write and let us know so we may rectify in any future reprint.

Except as permitted under U.S. Copyright Law, no part of this book may be reprinted, reproduced, transmitted, or utilized in any form by any electronic, mechanical, or other means, now known or hereafter invented, including photocopying, microfilming, and recording, or in any information storage or retrieval system, without written permission from the publishers.

For permission to photocopy or use material electronically from this work, please access www.copyright.com (http://www.copyright.com/) or contact the Copyright Clearance Center, Inc. (CCC), 222 Rosewood Drive, Danvers, MA 01923, 978-750-8400. CCC is a not-for-profit organization that provides licenses and registration for a variety of users. For organizations that have been granted a photocopy license by the CCC, a separate system of payment has been arranged.

Trademark Notice: Product or corporate names may be trademarks or registered trademarks, and are used only for identification and explanation without intent to infringe.

Visit the Taylor & Francis Web site at
http://www.taylorandfrancis.com

and the CRC Press Web site at
http://www.crcpress.com

Authors' affiliations

Amy Chang, OD, FAAO, FCOVD

Qualifications:

- State University of New York College of Optometry, New York, New York (2010)
- Residency in Acquired Brain Injury Rehabilitation at the State University of New York College of Optometry, New York, New York (2011)

Affiliations:

- Fellow of the College of Optometrists for Visual Development, Aurora, Ohio
- Fellow of the American Academy of Optometry, Orlando, Florida
- Developmental Optometrist of Hennepin County Medical Center, Traumatic Brain Injury Outpatient Clinic, Minneapolis, Minnesota

Steven E. Ritter, OD, FCOVD

Qualifications:

- State University of New York College of Optometry, New York, New York (1988)

Affiliations:

- Fellow of the College of Optometrists for Visual Development, Aurora, Ohio
- Assistant Clinical Professor of the State University of New York College of Optometry, New York, New York

Xiao Xi Yu, OD, FAAO

Qualifications:

- Pennsylvania College of Optometry at Salus University, Elkins Park, Pennsylvania (2010)
- Residency in Low Vision Rehabilitation at the State University of New York College of Optometry and Lighthouse International, New York, New York (2011)

Affiliations:

- Fellow of the American Academy of Optometry, Orlando, Florida
- Chief of Low Vision Service at West Los Angeles Veterans Health Administration, Los Angeles, California
- Assistant Professor at the Southern California College of Optometry, Marshall B. Ketchum University, Fullerton, California

Contents

Authors' disclaimer

The content in this book is for health-care professionals. It is not meant for the general consumer. The general consumer should not perform any of the activities discussed in this manual without the guidance of a trained health-care professional. Doing so may cause harm to their vision.

This is a guideline and manual for the optometric treatment of patients with traumatic brain injury. These therapy exercises are meant to be done under the guidance of an optometrist or an ophthalmologist, preferably one trained in vision rehabilitation. This manual lists many activities that legally require one of these two professionals to prescribe the treatments before they can be given to the patient. Specifically, treatment that involves accommodation lenses, prisms, and antisuppression can be harmful if it is performed on patients who are contraindicated for the exercise. For example, training antisuppression therapy on a patient who has anomalous retinal correspondence could result in the patient having intractable diplopia. This specific scenario is not common but is possible if treatment is not done under the supervision of an optometrist or an ophthalmologist.

Preface

This book came into existence when one of my therapists, Cherise March, told me that she would learn this material much faster if it was written down in a step-by-step fashion. I then realized there were no manuals available that discussed the treatment of patients with visual dysfunction after traumatic brain injury. There are manuals written mainly for the pediatric population, but a manual specifically focused in treating patients with TBI was nowhere to be found. Four years later, that excellent idea has finally turned into a published manual. In addition to flow sheets and worksheets, there are chapters that discuss theories and new treatments for TBI patients, as I found that many textbooks on this topic were lacking in practical applications. From my first position as the first neurooptometrist in the Department of Defense, seeing thousands of wounded soldiers in an active duty military hospital and working as a developmental optometrist at a level 1 trauma center in an inner-city hospital, there has been a broad patient base to draw experience from. I, of course, cannot take credit for my knowledge as it has been so graciously shared to me by many amazing professionals. First, I thank Dr. Allen Cohen and Dr. Neera Kapoor, my residency director and mentor, respectively. They are extremely distinguished doctors in the field of brain injury vision rehabilitation and have taught me so much in terms of diagnosis and treatment, as well as how to be a compassionate doctor. The therapy procedures that have been taught to me by Dr. Cohen and Dr. Kapoor comprise a very large portion of this manual. Second, I thank Dr. Steve Ritter and Dr. Shawn Yu for writing chapters in their areas of expertise; this manual could not have been complete without their work. I also thank all of the occupational therapists that I have had the sincere pleasure to work with; I absolutely believe a partnership between developmental optometry and occupational therapy is a positive one for our patients. And finally, I thank my husband, James, for his love and encouragement.

Please note that all exercises that can be given as a home exercise program (HEP) will be written in the language directed at the patient. All exercises that are for in-office purposes only will be written in the language directed at the therapist.

Dedication

This book is dedicated to all the military women and men who have served and continue to serve this country. I have had the privilege to be part of their rehabilitation. Your hard work, honor, and loyalty to our country continue to motivate me to grow in this profession. Thank you.

1

Philosophy of vision rehabilitation

Vision is a complex processing system that involves a lot more than just visual acuity, and being a complex system, it is useful to have a systematic approach to evaluate and treat visual deficits. This systematic approach is helpful in answering the question "what do we treat first" as sequencing does matter. If we view the visual system as a hierarchy where deficits in basic or foundational visual processing can adversely affect complex visual processing, we can easily see why it would be beneficial to address the foundational deficits first (see Figure 1.1).

VISUAL ACUITY AND VISUAL FIELD

The first aspect of vision is the simplest aspect of "seeing." Without having adequate visual acuity and visual field, there is a limit to what can be achieved with vision rehabilitation. This can be a major problem in patients who have traumatic optic neuropathy, hydrocephalous, posterior cerebral artery stroke resulting in hemianopia, and optic tract lesions, just to name a few. Rehabilitation is possible, but more challenging, and low vision will play a significant part in this patient's rehabilitation. Thankfully, this is by far the smaller percentage of patients who come in for evaluation. Significant decreased vision or visual field is uncommon in the mild–moderate traumatic brain injury (TBI) population. It is worth mentioning that when we are speaking of normal visual fields we are referring to peripheral visual sensitivity as testing with a static visual field instrument such as a Humphrey. Functional visual fields are frequently affected in mild–moderate TBI, and we will review that topic later on. With the mild–moderate TBI population, we are concerned with refractive

error. Small amounts of refractive error can make a huge difference in this population—the brain is injured, and with visually symptomatic patients, we know that the visual pathway connections are slowed (Ciuffreda et al. 2012), blur interpretation is decreased, and so small amounts of refractive errors are much more disabling than in a non-brain-injured individual. This is very important to keep in mind. Refractive error is also important in bottom-up visual processing as a correction at the "bottom" (see Figure 1.1)—visual acuity will affect everything else in the hierarchy; it will improve accommodation, fixation, pursuits, saccades, and binocularity. This is an important point to keep in mind.

Accommodation

Much like visual acuity, accurate and adequate accommodation is necessary for maintaining clear and comfortable vision (Leigh and Zee 2006, 345). Accommodation is dynamic and therefore is much more complex. The neuropathways are not completely understood, but it is important to know that accommodation is controlled by higher-order visual processes, in addition to the parasympathetic pathway.

Fixation

In the simplest form, it is the ability for the eye to maintain steady foveation of an object in space. The frontal eye field and rostral pole of the superior colliculus are the cortical and subcortical regions that control fixation (Leigh and Zee 2006, 291). Fixation is also a measurement of global attention; therefore, if a patient has poor attention, they will

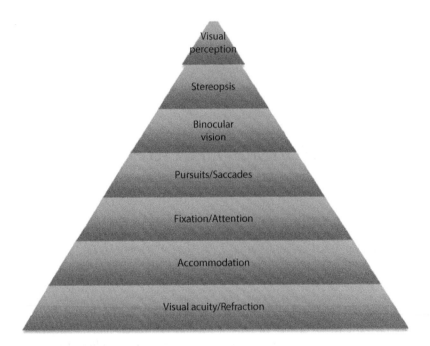

Figure 1.1 Visual hierarchy and therapy sequencing.

oftentimes have difficulty sustaining fixation on a visual task (Thompson and Amedee 2009, 20–26). Nystagmus is an obvious defect of fixation, where a steady fixation is absent and replaced with a back-and-forth movement. In patients with TBI, the nystagmus can be peripheral vestibular in nature such as in benign paroxysmal positional vertigo or central vestibular in nature arising from cerebellar or brainstem lesions (Leigh and Zee 2006, 673). It is important to address deficits of fixation early on in vision rehabilitation as pursuit and saccadic eye movements depend on accurate fixation.

Pursuit

Smooth-pursuit eye movements are utilized when tracking moving objects in an environment. The ability to execute accurate pursuits relies on a complex scheme where a movement of an object in space is perceived by the retina, which then travels from the lateral geniculate nucleus to the primary visual cortex (V1). From V1, the signal travels to the extra striate cortex and frontal eye fields where it then travels down to the cerebellum and projects to the brainstem premotor areas. Finally, signal arrives at the ocular motor neurons (cranial nerves 3, 4, and 6), where it results in a smooth-pursuit eye

movement (Leigh and Zee 2006, 203). In the TBI patient, addressing pursuit deficits can improve symptoms of sensitivity to visual motion. It is important to note that severe convergence disorders can also affect smooth pursuits and that if this is found upon examination, pursuit therapy should be performed monocularly to ensure that both eyes are able to perform the task before pursuing binocular therapy.

Saccades

Saccades are rapid eye movements that shift the center focus between successive points of fixation. Saccades are broken into many different types and can be classified into voluntary and involuntary saccades. Reflexive saccades are involuntary; they are generated to something unexpected in the environment, such as a loud sound or bright light. Reading is an example of voluntary saccades as they are made as part of purposeful behavior. Saccades are also very important for visual scan, which is necessary for seeing the gestalt when looking at a picture or taking in a new environment. The neurological pathway for saccades involves both cortical and subcortical areas. Excitatory burst neurons in the midbrain and pons generate the premotor commands for saccades. The cerebral cortex can trigger saccades via parallel descending pathway to the superior colliculus. Voluntary saccades depend on the frontal eye fields, and involuntary saccades depend on the parietal lobe to the superior colliculus. Finally, the cerebellum calibrates the saccade for accurate visual ocular motor movement. Injury or degeneration of the cerebellum will result in consistent hypermetric/hypometric saccades (Leigh and Zee 2006, 108–167). It is worth mentioning that adequate binocular vision is important for accurate saccades as well. If the patient has difficulty with coordinating their eyes and are not able to compute the three-dimensional location of the object, they are also going to have a lot of difficulty making an accurate saccade to the object and will likely make an over- or undershoot. Again if you are going to be performing a saccadic therapy technique in the setting of very poor binocularity, you would want to approach this therapy monocularly at first.

Binocular vision

Binocular vision is the ability for the two eyes to maintain bifoveal fixation of a single object of interest. If the eyes cannot perform this task, one will experience diplopia or suppression. Diplopia or double vision is usually very disturbing, so if the diplopia is not resolved within a certain period of time, the brain will suppress the vision of one eye. It is important to note that suppression is only under binocular viewing conditions. If either eye is occluded, there will not be suppression. Correcting for diplopia and suppression is an important step in neurovision rehabilitation as vergence eye movements and stereopsis cannot reliably occur with either of these conditions. Suppression is oftentimes difficult to recognize and is frequently missed in therapists who are not formally trained in neurovision rehabilitation. Red/green-based tests are best to use to detect suppression.

In addition to suppression, physiological diplopia is important as well. Physiological diplopia is a normal phenomenon where objects not within the area of fixation are seen as double. It is not just the absence of diplopia that indicates strong binocularity but the presence of physiological diplopia (pdipl). The general trend is that esotropes/esophores will tend to suppress pdipl proximal to the object being viewed, while exotropes/exophores will do the opposite. Without the proper pdipl feedback, the patient does not have the neuronal circuits to sustain vergence; if pdipl is not normalized upon completion of therapy, vergence deficits are more likely to regress.

BINOCULAR FUSION AND STEREOPSIS

Binocular fusion is the ability for the image of the object of interest to fall on corresponding retinal points of each eye and be perceived as a single image. Stereopsis is the three-dimensional perception of an object that occurs because each eye receives a slightly different image of an object.

VERGENCE

Vergence is a disconjugate eye movement, meaning the eyes are rotated in opposite directions, that is necessary to maintain binocular vision in the three-dimensional world. There are two main stimuli for vergence eye movements, the first is disparity-induced vergence, and this is when the new object of interest is at a different focal distance than the previous one. The new object falls onto noncorresponding retinal points, which causes diplopia; this drives the vergence system to make a movement to bring the new object onto corresponding retinal points and resolve the diplopia. The second stimuli for vergence is blur-induced vergence; the accommodative system is linked with the vergence system. For each diopter of accommodation, there is a set degree change of vergence. This relationship is referred to as the accommodative convergence to accommodation (AC/A) ratio. The normal AC/A ratio is 6, in which 6 diopters of convergence is exerted for every diopter increase in accommodation. This is an important concept as many binocular vision disorders arise from abnormally high or low AC/A ratios (Leigh and Zee 2006, 343–358).

The neurological pathway for convergence involves the midbrain, which houses the neurons involved specifically in the control of vergence; this then projects to the ocular motor neurons. There are also a number of cortical areas that contribute to vergence movements. The primary visual cortex contains neurons for stereopsis and vergence responses for small disparities. The middle temporal lobe and, important for perception of depth, the parietal lobe contribute to transforming visual signals from retinal to body-centered coordinates so that objects can be located in three-dimensional space. The frontal eye fields contain neurons that discharge for objects moving in depth. The cerebellum also plays a role in control of convergence eye movements as impaired convergence is often seen in patients with cerebellar lesions.

VISUAL PERCEPTION

Visual perception is its own category, but many of the concepts in visual perception are closely intertwined with lower visual processes. An example is visual attention and visual fixation. Visual fixation is a very basic process in which the subject has to stabilize their gaze on a target, while visual attention is a perceptual process that the mind has to focus on the object, which is challenged in a busy environment. Keeping in mind the parallels, let us delve into hierarchy of visual perception. At the basic level, we have visual attention. It came to be thought of as a three-step process. The first is disengaging the first object, the second is shifting of gaze to the new object location, and the third is to actively engage on the new object. Visual fixation and saccades are essential in visual attention. The next step is pattern recognition, which is the ability to identify the salient features of an object, or the gestalt. Aspects such as shape contour and color are all aspects of pattern recognition. And as with all hierarchies, visual attention is crucial in pattern recognition; inefficient attention will make identifying details challenging. Visual memory is the next component that involves recalling the image immediately after seeing it, as well is storing it in the memory to retrieve it later. The last component is visual cognition, which is the ability to mentally manipulate visual information and integrate it with other sense organs. This includes activities of everyday life such as making decisions and solving problems both in and out of the classroom (Warren 1993, 42).

TOP-DOWN VERSUS BOTTOM-UP APPROACH TO VISION REHABILITATION

Now that we have reviewed the visual hierarchy, it is time to discuss the two different pathways for treatment. In treating TBI patients, I have found that there are really two different groups of patients with one group responding best to the top-down approach and the second group responding best to the bottom-up approach. This distinction has been essential in effectively treating patients with TBI.

We will define top-down vision therapy as therapy that primarily uses the frontal cortex and visual attention to rehabilitate visual deficits. Bottom-up vision therapy is primarily sensory and subcortical based; this therapy utilizes the visual, vestibular, auditory, and somatosensory system to rehabilitate visual deficits.

Patients who benefit most from the top-down vision therapy approach are usually the less symptomatic group. There is not as much of an overload on their visual system. They typically are less light sensitive and many times are less aware that their symptoms are related to vision problems. These patients typically have normal distance binocular findings, accommodation and convergence are only mildly reduced, and oculomotor skills are very close to normal. For these patients, they need to improve the accuracy, latency, and endurance of their binocular, accommodative, and oculomotor skills. It is recommended to follow the sequencing of therapy as described in the therapy section.

Patients who benefit from bottom-up vision therapy are usually very symptomatic; they are easily overstimulated by light and sound. They also usually have symptoms of disequilibrium and imbalance. They are usually very disturbed by visual motion, such as watching cars pass on the road, or even a hand moving in front of them. Their visual ability fluctuates and is greatly influenced by outside factors such as fatigue, headaches, sleep, and stress. These patients often have reduced convergence and divergence ranges. These patients do not seem to respond as well to the top-down therapy approach as they usually feel a significant increase in symptoms with accommodation and convergence therapy. For these patients, tinted lenses, binasal occlusion, and yoked prism glasses are helpful treatment modalities. In neurovision rehabilitation, these patients benefit from sensory integration–type therapy, integrating their balance, vision, and auditory systems. Peripheral awareness therapy is also very helpful for these patients.

COMPONENTS FOR EFFECTIVE VISION THERAPY*

To be effective when treating patients with TBI, vision therapy techniques must incorporate the newly understood mechanisms of top-down visual processing and neuroplasticity. Cohen refers to five components of effective vision therapy: motivation, feedback, repetition, sensorimotor mismatch, and intermodal integration. Each component involves some degree of top-down processing. By incorporating these components into a vision therapy program, neuroplastic changes can be enhanced, resulting in a more effective treatment program. Each component is discussed in detail along with the associated neuroscience foundation.

Motivation/active participation

This is a conscious, goal-directed effort, which results in the activation of the prefrontal cortex to effect neuroplastic changes in the complex processing streams involved in visual perception. Motivation drives the patient to be an active participant in therapy, and understanding the goals and process of each procedure helps to sustain this level of participation at a therapeutic level. Studies have shown that prefrontal parietal integration resulted in the recovery of function in aphasics. Activation of the prefrontal cortex coupled with visually guided movement is the visual correlate to that study and is thought to promote recruitment and recovery of function.

Repetition

Repetition is the next component and is necessary for neuroplastic changes to occur. Kandel's research in neuroplasticity demonstrated that repeated stimulation of a neuron resulted in increased synaptic strength. He also found that repeated stimulation interspersed with periods of rest resulted in changes that lasted much longer than larger but less frequent periods of stimulation. The research that Kandel performed was on a simpler organism, the Aplysia; however, similar research performed on humans (with a much more complex neurological system) corroborates his findings.

Feedback

Feedback is the utilization of information to recalibrate and to refine encoded responses. The speed and accuracy of top-down processing is modulated and refined by sensory and motor feedback, such as auditory, visual, and proprioceptive cues. One excellent visual feedback mechanism is to use physiological diplopia in developing the sensorimotor tasks of triangulating the visual system to an area in space. Spatial working memory and accurate spatial localization are important in guiding the ocular motor system for convergence to a near object. The polarized vectogram is a good example of using this high-level feedback. By developing the awareness of physiological diplopia with a pointer, the patient learns to use physiological diplopia as feedback to guide and to confirm the location of the virtual projection within the spatial horopter. Auditory feedback can be introduced in many of the neurovision rehabilitator software (NVR) modules. In the visual-motor enhancer module, the patient maintains eye fixation on a designated letter that is displayed on a rotating pegboard. When the patient guides the remote control outside of the designated letter, the patient will hear a sharp beeping tone that will continue until the patient guides the remote control back inside the designated letter. This top-down visual-motor adjustment, which is initiated by auditory cues, is an example of an auditory feedback procedure.

Motor match to a sensory mismatch

Performance in the multisensory world requires input from many areas, including the visual cortex, premotor cortex, motor cortex, basal ganglia, cerebellum, and brainstem. All of these areas relay information to the parietal cortex. Subsequently, the parietal cortex relays this information to the different visual processing pathways, including the parietal–prefrontal and parietal–premotor pathways. The parietal and cerebellar regions are

---

* This section is excerpted from Chang, A., Kapoor, N., and Cohen, A.H. 2013. Top-down visual framework for optometric vision therapy for those with traumatic brain injury. *Optom Vis Perform.* 1:48–53.

activated in the initial error-correction phase. Since the visual pathways that originate in the parietal cortex are affected by TBI, the ability to make these rapid adaptations is diminished. Therefore, one of the deficits evident in those with TBI is reduced speed of retrieval of these learned, visually guided motor skills, which may contribute to the disequilibrium that those with TBI experience. Loading visual therapy procedures with filters, yoked prism, stereoscopic cards used in a stereoscope, and various lens combinations can manipulate the visual input. Then, with appropriate feedback modalities, the patient guides their motor response to this input, which is important in enhancing sensorimotor recalibration.

Multisensory integration (intermodal)

As discussed earlier, TBI often affects pathways associated with the parietal and prefrontal lobes, resulting in reduced speed of processing. As a result of the reduced speed and inefficiency of the parietal lobe and associated processing streams, those with TBI often feel overwhelmed and disoriented, especially when there are unpredictable visual changes, smells, and sounds in their environment. By systematically loading vision therapy procedures with balance, vision, motor, and auditory inputs, the speed of visual information processing may be enhanced. Any therapy procedure that incorporates the use of a balance board and metronome with ocular motility may be used to develop this important neuroprocessing skill.

An example of a procedure incorporating this concept is the ocular vestibular integrator module of the NVR. The patient views a large projection of multiple targets and is instructed to fixate a central point while being aware of, but not distracted by, peripheral targets. As the targets located peripherally light up, the patient experiences the awareness of the spatial position of the target. This awareness of the peripheral spatial position of the target is utilized to direct the patient's eyes to the target. Once their eyes are on the target, the patient attempts to eliminate the target by using their visual system to guide their hand, which is holding a remote control device. The accuracy of the elimination is

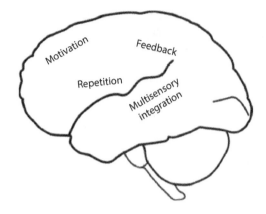

Figure 1.2 Components for effective vision therapy.

confirmed by an auditory beep. This procedure can be made more challenging by adding distractors, which serve as bottom-up stimuli, that appear at random times. Improved performance enhances peripheral awareness, visual attention, accurate visually guided saccades, and visual-motor control, all of which are important in rebalancing top-down and bottom-up visual processing.

A more general guideline to procedures that incorporate multisensory integration is the use of multiple Post-it notes, labeled with either numbers or letters, which are randomly placed on a wall. These act as both central and peripheral targets, meaning that the patient first has to find the designated character with their peripheral vision and then make an accurate saccade to that Post-it and fixate on it with their central vision. To make this more challenging, the patient can be instructed to use a laser pointer in order to use eye-directed (goal-directed top-down) motor movement to place the laser directly on the designated Post-it note. The OEP clinical curriculum has standardized the central peripheral saccades and flashlight pointing procedures that incorporate the same concepts listed earlier. Other instruments that can be used are the Wayne Saccadic Fixator, stick ups, and the space localizer. Adding a balance board further integrates the vestibular system to this procedure, and having the patient wait a specified number of metronome beats before moving on to the next target allows auditory integration (Figure 1.2).

REFERENCES

Ciuffreda, K.J. Yadav, N.K, and Ludlam, D.P. 2012. Effect of binasal occlusion on the visual evoked potential in mild traumatic brain injury. *Brain Inj*. 27:41–47.

Leigh, H. and Zee, P. 2006. *The Neurology of Eye Movements*, 4th edn. New York: Oxford University Press.

Thompson, T.L. and Amedee, R. 2011. Vertigo: A review of common peripheral and central vestibular disorders. *Ochsner J*. 9:20–26.

Warren, M. 1993. A hierarchical model for evaluation and treatment of visual perceptual dysfunction in adult acquired brain injury, part 1. *Am J Occup Ther*. 47:55–66.

2

Evaluation and treatment of the mild/mod TBI patient

The first step to evaluating the traumatic brain injury (TBI) patient is obtaining a careful case history. The date of the injury, severity, and type of injury are important, as well as a full medical, surgical, and ocular history. Sometimes, the patient will have a long list of visual complaints and other times they may only have a few. It is helpful to have patients elaborate on vague symptoms as having a clear understanding of their symptoms is important in the diagnosis and treatment of the patient. A symptoms survey is recommended as oftentimes patients are unaware that certain symptoms are related to their vision, for example, difficulty reading, and disequilibrium. What follows is the post-traumatic vision survey (see Appendix) that the author uses for their patients. Then, a list of the tests that are performed as part of a comprehensive neurooptometric evaluation is given.

EXAMINATION

The following will not be described in detail as they are straightforward and no modifications are needed for the TBI population:

- Distance and near acuities
- Distance and near cover test
- Color vision
- Stereo testing
- Intraocular pressure
- Confrontational visual field
- Anterior and posterior segment

Fixation/pursuits/saccades

Have the patient fixate on a target approximately 18″ from their nose. A good target would be a Wolff Wand or something similar. There is a standard grading system for ocular motility, called the NSUCO oculomotor test; however, it is geared more for the pediatric population. Another more simple grading system is a scale 1–4, where 4 represents a normal finding and 1 represents a severely abnormal finding. In addition to the scale, it would be helpful to describe the deficits that are present.

1. *Fixation ability*: Have the patient fixate on a target for 10 seconds. This should be done monocularly. Record any fixation intrusions or latent nystagmus.
2. *Pursuit ability*: Have the patient make a full rotation clockwise and counterclockwise. Record any refixations, in which direction, and any gaze-evoked or end-gaze nystagmus.
3. *Saccadic ability*: Have the patient jump between two targets, from midline to right, from midline to left, midline to superior field, midline to inferior field. Indicate if there are hypometric or hypermetric saccades and in which direction they were seen.

Free space vertical and horizontal phoria at distance

This is important to perform as oftentimes the binocular dysfunction is present at distance as well.

To perform the vertical phoria, use a single 20/30 letter and hold a 6-diopter base-in prism in front of the left eye and ask the patient if they see double; if so, then ask them if the letters lined up like headlights on a car. If it is, you are done with this test and can record "iso"; if not, place the vertical prism bar in front of their right eye until the patient reports the letters are aligned, and then record the finding.

To perform the horizontal phoria, use the same single 20/30 letter and hold a 4-diopter base-down prism in front of the left eye; ask the patient if the letters line up like buttons on a shirt. If so, you are done with this test and can record ortho; if not, introduce the horizontal prism in front of their right eye until the letters are aligned and then record the finding.

Free space horizontal phoria at near

This can be performed in the same manner as the distance using a 20/30 letter at near. It is helpful to perform Maddox rod testing at near to uncover subtle vertical deviations.

Dynamic Worth 4 Dot

This is an important test to determine whether there is any suppression. This test is performed at multiple distances to rule out any intermittent suppression. The patient should be seated and be wearing their correction and red and green glasses. Start by holding the Worth 4 Dot at 4′ away and ask them if they see 4 dots and if they are lined up like a diamond. Then, start walking further away and ask them if it changes. If it does not, then record flat fusion at distance; if it does, then record the finding whether it is suppression or eso/exo diplopia. To test for suppression at the near range, move toward the patient and evaluate at 16″. You can then move the Worth 4 Dot closer to the patient and measure their ability to sustain flat fusion at even closer distances; oftentimes, there will be an exo diplopia response at near; record this break and recovery.

Fixation dot with head shake

Have patient wear R/G glasses and look at a fixation dot on projector, and ask the patient how many dots they see. Are they overlapping? If not, record, eso/exo/vertical diplopia. Then, have patient shake head from side to side at a rate of 1–2 rotations/second and ask them what happens; does the dots split? Exo? Eso?

Or unsteady (retinal slip)? This is a measure of VOR (vestibular ocular reflex) and binocular stability at distance; if this finding is abnormal, the patient may experience unsteady vision with head movements. Dynamic acuity can also be measured at distance by asking the patient to view a line of letters two lines better than their best corrected distance visual acuity. The examiner will stand behind the patient and move their head 20°–30° from midline at a rate of two cycles per second. If the patient is unable to read the letters on the chart, this is considered a positive result (Dannenbaum et al. 2009, 268).

Vergence ranges convergence and divergence at distance and at near

This is important for determining their range of visual comfort. Normal vergence ranges represent binocular stability, reduced ranges in one direction represent a binocular dysfunction, and reduced ranges in both directions represent binocular instability. It is best to use a vertical line for testing as this allows for the distinction between blurry versus true diplopia. Record the prism of the first blur, then break (diplopia) and finally recovery (when they are able to regain single vision). It is recommended to perform this test in free space with a prism bar versus in a phoropter. The phoropter blocks out much of the patient's peripheral vision and so it is a more artificial environment.

Near point of convergence

This is usually performed with a single letter or a line of letters approximately 20/30 in size on a tongue depressor. The patient is asked to state when the letter is double. The tongue depressor is then moved away from the patient, and they are asked to state when the letter is single again. Record the distance from the patient's nose of the break and recovery. Note if either eye consistently turned out and if the patient had diplopia awareness when their eyes were not aligned. This test is usually performed twice to determine consistency of response and to determine whether the patient worsens upon repetition.

Near point of convergence with red lens and pen light

Hold the red lens in front of the right eye and pen light in line with the patient's nose starting at 16" away, and slowly bring in the penlight toward the patient until they report two lights. Record this distance as the break. Bring the light away from the patient until they report the light becomes single; this is the recovery. If the patient does not report the light becoming double record this as "to the nose." This measures the patient's convergence without accommodation. Patients who are relying more on their accommodation to sustain convergence may perform significantly worse with this testing.

Retinoscopy

This is performed in the standard manner, but it is important to note that there are latent hyperopic patients who complain of blurry vision at distance and may have 20/20 unaided acuity, so it is important to perform this on every patient.

Refraction

This is again performed in the standard manner, but important to note that many TBI patients have accommodative spasm or infacility. To obtain the most accurate results, do not fog the patient more than 0.50 diopters. If the patient reports the letters are coming in and out of focus, it may be helpful to increase the size of the letters by two lines, have the patient close their eyes, and take deep breaths to relax before continuing. If the patient cannot be corrected to 20/20 and you do not suspect ocular disease or amblyopia, it is usually necessary to cycloplege the patient.

Fused cross-cylinder/monocular estimation method/plus build-up

Again there are no modifications necessary to perform this test; it is important to perform at least two of these three tests to determine whether there is a lead or lag of accommodation and whether there is a need for a near add.

Negative relative accommodation/positive relative accommodation

This is a helpful test to determine the severity of the accommodative deficits.

Minus lens amplitude

This test determines their maximum accommodation. As a rule to sustain accommodation, the patient needs twice their accommodative demand. For example, if the patient has a working distance of 16″, they required 2.5 diopters of accommodation for that task; therefore, they would need a minimum of 5 diopters of accommodation. Accommodation is age dependent. Hofstetter's equation can be used to determine the normative value for the patient. There are multiple methods to determine accommodative amplitude with minus lens to be the best method as it controls for the size of the target.

Pupillary testing

In addition to the standard pupillary testing, it is important to test the sustained pupillary constriction ability. The presence of an "alpha-omega pupil," which is a pupil that fails to constrict, or may constrict but fail to hold the constriction to light, indicates autonomic fatigue; the faster the dilation in the presence of the light source, the smaller the functional field. A normal pupil should constrict and hold the constriction for at least 15 seconds (Wallace 2009, 73).

Visual field testing

Traditional automated perimetry is recommended in patients suspected of having optic nerve or tract injury and patients who have positive findings on brain imaging that would raise suspicion of hemianopic or quadranopic visual field defects. Full-field testing can be performed if the patient reports subjective visual field loss outside of the central 30°. Kinetic visual field testing is another test that can be helpful for measuring the functional visual field; this can be done if the patient has difficulty progressing in neurovision rehab or if they are very symptomatic and the testing does not reveal significant deficits. Kinetic testing is best done with a campimeter, with four different stimuli, white, red, green, and blue (Wallace 2009, 73).

15 Prism diopter yoked prism evaluation

This test provides insight into how the patient processes visual information both on a subcortical and cortical level (Zelinsky 2007, 87). To perform the test, the patient is instructed to walk in a straight line while wearing 15 prism diopter yoked prism. This test is repeated with prisms yoked, up, down, left, and right. A railing or gait belt should be provided for this patient for safety measures as some patients may lose their balance. What follows are possible patient responses and their interpretation.

If the patient rotates their body, leans forward, backward, left, or right, reaches out their arms to steady themselves, or complains of being dizzy or feels as if they are falling, this represents difficulty with ambient visual processing on a subcortical level.

If the patient describes distortions in their environment or perceives objects as being slanted, closer or farther, bigger or smaller, this represents difficulty with ambient visual processing on a cortical level.

If one or two of the prism directions are significantly easier for the patient to ambulate, repeat the testing with 2 prism diopters yoked in those directions. Consider prescribing 2-diopter yoked prism in the direction the patient was most comfortable with. Oftentimes, retesting pursuit, saccade, and phoria measurements with the tentative yoked prisms in place can improve the above deficits, further validating the need for the prismatic correction.

ANALYZING THE DATA

There are many textbooks and references that discuss the diagnosis of different binocular disorders in the non-TBI population. We will not review those concepts; instead, we will focus on the most common disorders seen in this population.

Pursuit/saccadic dysfunction

If either of these deficits is found, neurovision rehabilitation is recommended to address these deficits.

Accommodative insufficiency/ infacility

This is diagnosed if the patient has reduced negative relative accommodation (NRA)/positive relative accommodation (PRA), monocular accommodative amplitude, or accommodative facility. This can be treated with near-prescription glasses and/or neurovision rehabilitation.

Binocular instability

The patient has decreased convergence and divergence ranges, which can be diagnosed at distance, near or both. This is best treated with neurovision rehabilitation. It is helpful to perform kinetic visual field testing on patients with binocular instability, as they are more likely to have constricted kinetic visual field. Treating the constricted visual field with peripheral awareness exercises and/or syntonic phototherapy can be useful. Binasal occlusion can also be helpful.

Convergence insufficiency

The patient has an exophoria that is greater at near, the base-in range is normal or close to normal, and the base-out range is reduced. The patient also has a decreased near point of convergence. This is best treated with neurovision rehabilitation.

Intermittent exotropia

The patient has a larger degree of exophoria and has a deviated eye under associated conditions (meaning neither eye is occluded). The patient may report intermittent diplopia. This can be treated with yoked prisms and neurovision rehabilitation.

Convergence excess

The esophoria is greater at near, with normal or near-normal convergence ranges, and deficient near-divergence ranges. This can be treated with near-prescription glasses and/or neurovision rehabilitation.

Divergence insufficiency

The esophoria is greater at distance with reduced distance divergence range. The patient will often report diplopia at a distance. This can be treated with prisms at distance and/or neurovision rehabilitation.

Divergence excess

This is rarely seen in the TBI population and likely represents a long-standing binocular dysfunction. These patients have an exophoria that is greater at distance than near. This can be treated with neuro-vision rehabilitation.

Suppression

Not a separate diagnosis, but important to consider in the assessment and plan. This should be treated with neurovision rehabilitation before beginning binocular therapy.

Photosensitivity

A very prevalent symptom within the TBI population. This can be treated with tinted lenses.

Transitions: Extra-active type, which are tinted indoors and darken outdoors, work best
15% blue tint: Indoor use, computer use, night-time driving.
15% blue blocker tint: Yellow tint that some find helpful for computer work and nighttime driving.
Anifra tint (12% blue-green tint): For indoor use.
Wrap around polarized sunglasses: For outdoor use.

Visual midline shift syndrome

Visual midline shift syndrome is a term developed by Dr. William Padula. It describes a change in visual processing that can occur after a neurological event. He describes it as the ambient visual process changing its concept of midline usually away from the neurologically affected side (Padula 1996, 165).

This is mainly treated with yoked prisms.

Deficit of ambient visual processing

Ambient visual processing, also known as the dorsal stream, is responsible for processing visual motion, and where the patient is in respect to their environment. Ambient vision interacts with other senses such as vestibular and somatosensory to determine spatial orientation and posture. When a patient has a deficit in their ambient visual processing, they will experience symptoms of disorientation, nausea, and imbalance (Committee on Vision 1985).

There are many treatment options, including tinted lenses, yoked prisms, binasal occlusion, and neurovision rehabilitation.

REFERENCES

Committee on Vision, National Research Council. 1985. *Emergent Techniques For Assessment Of Visual Performance*. Washington, DC: National Academies Press.

Dannenbaum, E., Paquet, N., Chilingaryan, G., and Fung, J. 2009. Clinical evaluation of dynamic visual acuity in subjects with unilateral vestibular hypofunction. *Otol Neurotol.* 30(3):368–372.

Padula, W. 1996. Post trauma vision syndrome and visual midline shift syndrome. *Neurorehabilitation.* 6:165–171. [Online.]

Wallace, L.B. 2009. The theory and practice of syntonic phototherapy: A review. *J Optom Vis Dev.* 40:73–81.

Zelinsky, D. 2007. Neuro-optometric diagnosis, treatment, and rehabilitation following traumatic brain injuries: A brief overview. *Phys Med Rehabil Clin North Am.* 18:87–107.

3

Guide to therapist evaluation and treatment of the mild–moderate traumatic brain injury patient

A therapist can perform a neuroocular screening on a patient with traumatic brain injury. What follows is a list of screening tests that can be performed:

VISUAL ACUITY SCREEN

- Test each eye singly (monocular) and both together (binocular).
- Snellen acuity chart—for far distance. Patient stands or sits with toes behind tape mark on floor (10, from chart). If patient is sitting, move chart down to patient's eye level.
- Rosenbaum pocket screen—for near vision. The smallest print that they can read >50% of the letters correctly is the level of acuity that is recorded.

FIXATION/PURSUITS/SACCADES

Please refer to the optometry evaluation as it can be performed the same way.

KING–DEVICK TEST

This is a test to measure the speed and accuracy of saccadic eye movements specifically for reading. This test is available for purchase from a number of different vendors. This test is normed for from age 6 to adult.

COVER TEST

To determine whether there is ocular misalignment, perform a cover/uncover test.

- First step is to find a fixation target: If the double vision is at distance, find a distance target at 10′ or further away; if the double vision is at near, hold the target 16″ away from the patient's nose.
- The target size is relatively important. It should be large enough for the patient to be able to see relatively clearly, but small enough to keep the patient's fixation steady. A letter is usually a good target to use.
- By instructing the patient to keep their eyes on the target, you will take an occluder (or your hand) and cover the left eye and pay attention to the right eye (the eye that is not being covered); if there is movement seen, this may be an eye turn, which can indicate ocular misalignment. If there is no movement, uncover the left eye and repeat, this time covering the right eye, and observe the left eye. Always observe the eye that is not being covered.
- You may want to repeat this test two to three times depending on the cooperation of the patient. If you consistently see one eye turn in, out, up, or down (it has to always be the same direction), then the patient's double vision is caused by an ocular misalignment.

- Turn: In (exo), out (eso), up (hypo), down (hyper).
- To perform an alternating cover test to determine whether there is a heterophoria, perform the test the same way, but this eye alternately covers each eye, and look for movement of the eye as you are uncovering it. The descriptions are as listed earlier.

NEAR POINT OF CONVERGENCE

Move a target from arm's length in midline toward the bridge of the nose. Observe to see whether the eyes move symmetrically through the full range. If one eye moves away from the target and the patient does not report double vision, this patient has suppression. See Chapter 2 for more details of this test.

WORTH 4 DOT

Make sure the patient wears their prescription glasses for this test (if applicable). Have the patient put on red/green glasses. Hold up the Worth 4 Dot (W4D), 2′ from the patient at their eye level and push the switch up to turn it on. Ask the patient how many dots they see. Record this result. Then, slowly move the W4D away from the patient to about 10′ and ask if it changes; record any changes they report. Then, return to 2′ away and bring the W4D slowly closer to the patient (up to 6″ away) and ask if it changes; record any changes they report.

Interpretation:

- *4 dots: Flat fusion*—This means there is no suppression and the eyes are aligned.
- *3 dots (green)*—Right eye suppression.
- *2 dots (red)*—Left eye suppression.
- *5 dots*—Diplopia.

CLOWN VECTOGRAM RANGES

- This test can detect convergence and divergence deficits at near. It is important to note that there are issues with the sensitivity of this test, meaning patients with convergence and divergence deficits could test normal.

- This test requires the use of a clown vectogram, polarized glasses (which is included with the vectogram) and holder, both of which can be purchased through Bernell.
- The patient should wear their spectacle correction (if applicable), and specifically their reading correction (if applicable), and be seated approximately 18″ away from the vectogram, and it should be at their eye level.
- The therapist should have the patient put on the polarized glasses and set the vectogram up so that only the "@" symbol is visible on the bottom of the vectogram.
- The therapist should separate the two slides, moving the front slide over to the right and back slide to the left; the numbers should now be appearing in the bottom of the vectogram. Instruct the patient to report when they see two sets of clowns. Then, slowly move the slides closer together until the patient reports the clown becomes single. Record the number where they reported seeing two, and number where they were able to see one again. This is their convergence range.
- This test should be repeated, but this time the front slide will be moved over to the left and back slide to the right. The letters will appear on the bottom of the vectogram; this represents their divergence range. There are no normative data on this test; from clinical experience, the norm for convergence is 25, and divergence is H, and poor recovery (the second number or letter) can also represent a deficit.

ACCOMMODATIVE FACILITY (IF OPTOMETRIST OR OPHTHALMOLOGIST IS ON STAFF IN YOUR OFFICE AND IS OVERSEEING YOUR TREATMENT)

- This test is to measure the focusing flexibility of the patient. This test requires the use of accommodative flipper, ±2.00 for patients age 5–35 and ±1.50 for patients 35–45. This test is not typically performed on patients who are >45 years of age due to natural decline in accommodation.

- The patient holds reading material at 16″ away from their eyes. This reading material should be approximately 20/30 in size.
- The therapist instructs the patient to hold one side of the lens up to their eyes and let the therapist know when the letters are clear or readable. The patient then flips the lens to the other side and repeats the same thing.
- The therapist keeps track of the testing time (1 minute) and how many cycles the patient was able to complete within the time period.
- The test is performed monocularly and then binocularly; the norms are 11 cycles per minute monocular and 8 cycles per minute binocular.

4

How to prescribe lenses and prisms

REFRACTIVE CORRECTION

A standard optometric refraction should be performed on a patient with traumatic brain injury (TBI). In general, TBI patients benefit from even small refractive corrections. If the patient has ambient visual processing deficits, prescribing low hyperopic prescriptions can allow for better comfort and more stable ambient processing (Zelinsky 2010, 852). Cycloplegic refractions are necessary for patients who cannot correct to 20/20 where you do not expect ocular disease or amblyopia to be the source. If there are significant fluctuations during refraction, this may also be an appropriate additional test. When prescribing near-vision glasses, it is helpful to remember that less is more. Patients with TBI often have reduced accommodative facility and will have difficulty relaxing their accommodation as well as increasing their accommodation. The best way to determine whether the proposed add will benefit the patient is to trial frame the patient with it. Note that most near-vision corrections for non-presbyopic patients are between +0.50 and +0.75 diopters.

PRISMS AND OPHTHALMIC TREATMENT FOR BINOCULAR DISORDERS

Prisms are commonly used in the TBI population and can be used as compensating or yoked prism. Compensating prism is often used for task-specific activities such as reading, while yoked prism is used to restore imbalances between the vision and balance systems on a subcortical level (Zelinsky 2010, 852).

CONVERGENCE INSUFFICIENCY

In patients with convergence insufficiency, base-in prism is the most frequent prism applied. There are several ways to determine the amount of prism necessary. Sheard's criterion is an excellent reference point. Sheard's criterion is an equation as follows:

Prism needed = 2/3 (Phoria) − 1/3 (Compensating fusional vergence)

The best way to implement this into an exam is to create a spreadsheet that has the Sheard's formula built in. This can eliminate manual calculation as a trial frame with the tentative prism will be helpful especially with patients who also have reduced base-in ranges.

BASIC EXOPHORIA

Patients who also have significant exophoria and reduced base-out range at distance will benefit from base-in prism full time. If base-in prism is only prescribed at near, every time the patient takes off the glasses to look at far distance, they will have a more difficult time diverging to the distance target. Prescribing full-time base-in prism for these patients will allow for more visual comfort and an easier time transitioning from near to far, and vice versa. A rule of thumb is, first, never prescribe more than the amount of deviation at distance (>4-diopter prism). Performing a red lens test at distance with the white dot on the projector will usually elicit crossed diplopia, which then base-in prism can be added until the diplopia is resolved. Yoked prisms are another option. Trial of 2-diopter base-down yoked prism is recommended. Remeasuring phoria and convergence as well as asking the patient for feedback can determine whether this is beneficial.

BINOCULAR INSTABILITY

For patients who have significantly decreased base-in ranges as well as base-out ranges or patients without a significant near exophoria, base-in prism may not be of much benefit. It is best to avoid prescribing base-in prism to patients who have an ortho or eso fixation disparity. These patients respond well to binasal occlusion or yoked prism.

CONVERGENCE EXCESS

Base-out prism is rarely prescribed for patients with convergence excess (CE). Plus lenses are the first treatment option. Findings to support plus lenses are age, fused cross cylinder, balance between negative relative accommodation (NRA) and positive relative accommodation (PRA), monocular estimation method, and AC/A ratio. These techniques will not be reviewed as they are easily found in other optometric literature. It is best to prescribe conservatively in cases where the patient has a lead of accommodation and discourage prescribing more than +1.50 on pre-presbyopes as most patients in this category spend a great deal of time on the computer, which is a greater working distance and less accommodative demand. Remember that more plus also narrows the depth of field and focus.

BINASAL OCCLUSION

Binasal occlusion is a method of partial covering of the visual field of the two eyes in which a section of the nasal visual field is occluded for each eye. By blocking parts of the field that is seen by both eyes, binasal occlusion reduces the visual stress that would be caused by over convergence (think of the strings intersecting in front of the bead). It also seems to be helpful for accommodative excess as it decreases the overconvergence component of that cycle. These patients also happen to complain of difficulty with visual motion and overstimulation in busy visual environments (Ciuffreda et al. 2013, 41). Binasal occlusion also

improves peripheral visual processing by discouraging esoposture and encouraging peripheral processing since objects that are located to the right can only be fixated by the right eye and those located to the left only by the left eye. To summarize, I would consider binasal occlusion on patients with convergence excess (esophoria and/or reduced base-in ranges), binocular instability (reduced base-in and base-out ranges), and accommodative excess patients.

YOKED PRISM

Yoked prisms can be used to improve patient's symptoms of dizziness or unsteadiness. Depending on which direction the prism is yoked, the light entering the eyes through the prism is bent as it is received by the retina. The light is then converted to electrical signals and can travel through a non-damaged area of the brain, improving patient's symptoms and eliciting a more favorable response (Zelinsky 2007, 87).

TREATMENT: NEUROVISION REHABILITATION

Neurovision rehabilitation is the main focus of this guide, and Chapters 5 through 9 have detailed flow sheets for designing the treatment plan for patients. These chapters also have detailed instructions on how to perform each therapy procedure.

NEUROVISION REHABILITATION TROUBLESHOOTING

As with all treatments, there are times when the patient does not seem to continue to make progress. What follows are the common obstacles that occur.

Top five roadblocks that occur in therapy

1. *Accommodation*: Sometimes, the patient's accommodation system is overlooked because they may have a more obvious binocular deficit such as a strabismus. There are many patients who have seemingly plateaued in binocular therapy because an underlying accommodative

deficit was not addressed. The best way to avoid this roadblock is to perform accommodative testing at the evaluation.

2. *Suppression*: Suppression is also an elusive roadblock to therapy; it can be present at only one working distance and can be intermittent. Physiological diplopia (pdipl) can be evaluated through the Brock's string exercise. Remember there are two main vergence symptoms; patients who rely heavily on accommodative convergence may have poor disparity vergence, and disparity vergence requires the presence of pdipl.

3. *Training both fusional ranges*: If a patient with convergence insufficiency returned for follow-up and was very symptomatic, it is most likely because the patient now had reduced base-in ranges. Making sure that both fusional ranges are trained will prevent this from happening. Jump ductions are important and so is the technique base-in minus, base-out plus.

4. *Dynamic vergence*: In the natural world, vergence eye movements are rarely isolated, vergence eye movements usually occur with a pursuit or saccadic eye movement. Incorporating saccade and pursuit eye movements with vergence activity will help the patient improve their visual stamina. Integrating head movement, multiple Brock's strings, or prism with tracking activities are all ways in which to train dynamic vergence.

5. *Saccades*: Patients should slow down when performing saccadic therapy. Slowing it down engages their visual attention to drive their saccades, instead of motor cues, that is, they will naturally use their finger or a laser pointer to guide their eyes where to look, but it should be the other way around; therefore have the patient find the target with their eyes first and then bring their finger or laser pointer to the target.

6. *Peripheral awareness*: If the patient has poor peripheral visual field awareness, they will have difficulty progressing in vision rehab. Performing a kinetic visual field as described in Chapter 2 can confirm your suspicions. Consider plus lenses, binasal occlusion, base-in prism, and/or syntonic phototherapy to treat this issue before continuing with vision rehab.

REFERENCES

Ciuffreda, K., Yadav, N.K., and Ludlam, D.P. 2013. Effect of binasal occlusion on the visual-evoked potential in mild traumatic brain injury. *Brain Inj.* 27:41–47.

Zelinsky, D.G. 2007. Neuro-optometric diagnosis, treatment and rehabilitation following traumatic brain injuries: A brief overview. *Phys Med Rehabil Clin N Am.* 18:87–107.

Zelinsky, D.G. 2010. Brain injury rehabilitation: Cortical and subcortical interfacing via retinal pathways. *PM R.* 2:852–857.

5

Evaluation and treatment of the severe traumatic brain injury patient

The examination of patients with severe traumatic brain injury (TBI) involves a different testing from that of patients with mild to moderate TBI. It does challenge the clinician to be particularly familiar with neuroanatomy. The differences will be described next.

HISTORY

In the examination of the severe TBI patient, history is even more important. Many times especially during the acute phase, the patient is often not going to be in the best cognitive or psychological state to be the best historian. This can be obtained by the hospital staff (if you are examining bedside) or the patient's family members. Information that would be helpful to have are MRI/CT scans of the head and/or report, neurologist/neurosurgeon reports, neuropsychology reports, and hospital discharge paper work. The neuroimaging is especially important as it will reveal the severity of the injury and the cortical and subcortical areas that are affected.

DEFINITIONS

Contusion: "Bruising" of brain tissue occurs in 20%–30% of severe brain injuries, can decline mental function, and is likely to heal on its own.

Infarct: This is usually not in TBI, but is very common in ischemic strokes and blockage in blood vessel supplying blood to the brain. This results in death of the surrounding tissue; they vary in their severity. One of the most common infarcts in cerebrovascular disease is of the posterior cerebral artery (PCA) that supplies the occipital lobe. Infarct on one side of the PCA results in a contralateral homonymous hemianopia (HH). Ischemic strokes usually have the least chance of resolution of the HH.

Intracranial hemorrhage: This can occur from a stroke or TBI; the hemorrhage occurs within the brain tissue. This is a serious medical emergency because it results in increased intracranial pressure.

Cerebral hypoxia: Decreased oxygen to the brain can be focal or diffuse. If severe enough, it can result in permanent severely decreased brain function.

AREAS TO PAY ATTENTION TO

Frontal lobe: In severe TBI, there is often frontal lobe dysfunction. This can be observed as difficulty maintaining fixation, difficulty initiating, and following moving targets (smooth pursuits).

Temporal lobe: Temporal lobe injury can result in superior quadrantanopia and will usually be associated with auditory/language processing difficulty (aphasia).

Parietal lobe: Can result in inferior quadrantanopia if the right hemisphere visual neglect is possible.

Occipital lobe: Occipital lobe injury usually results in an HH.

Cerebellum: This *can* result in balance difficulty, nystagmus, convergence insufficiency, and divergence insufficiency.

EXAMINATION

Distance acuities/near acuities: Attempt visual acuity testing when possible. Possible decreases in visual acuity are large compressions chiasmal/prechiasmal. Traumatic optic neuropathy and bilateral posterior cerebral artery infarcts. Even with these possibilities, decreased visual acuity is still not that common since the injury usually occurs post chiasmal; therefore, it is most likely that central vision is preserved. If patient participation is poor and there is difficulty determining decreased visual acuity, consider patching the "good" eye during the exam and see whether there is any resistance from the patient.

Fixation (monocular)/pursuits/saccades: Testing is the same as with mild–moderate TBI. Fixation is an active process, which is a function of visual attention, and requires frontal lobe and cerebellar/brainstem function.

Pursuits: Cerebellum/brainstem, looking for refixations, gaze-evoked nystagmus, and noncomitancy.

Saccades: Most complex, cortical function as well as brainstem, looking for slowness and overshoot/undershoots.

Distance cover test/near cover test and ocular alignment testing: Noncomitancy that will point you to a cranial nerve (CN) palsy; cranial nerve 4 and 6 palsies are very common.

Near point of convergence: Important to perform as cerebellar and midbrain lesions will show decreased convergence.

Retinoscopy: This is an objective test to determine their refractive status.

Refraction: This test should be performed if possible.

Automated and confrontational visual field: Important to perform visual field as defects are quite common in severe TBI.

Pupils: This is an important test as pupillary function can reveal asymmetry in visual function; a patient with bilateral poorly reactive pupils can indicate increased intracranial pressure or brainstem compression (Chen et. al. 2011, 82).

Ophthalmoscopy: Important to rule out increased intracranial pressure (papilledema), traumatic optic neuropathy, or other ocular trauma.

SUPPLEMENTARY TESTS

15-Diopter yoked prism evaluation

This test can be performed the same way it is described for mild–moderate TBI patients if the patient can tolerate it. Otherwise, it can be modified for patients with significant gait disturbances. Instead of 15-diopter prism, 4-diopter yoked prisms can be used. Trial the patient with the prisms in all four directions and determine whether there is one or two directions that seem to be of the most benefit. Consider prescribing 2-diopter prism in the direction that was the most beneficial. If the patient is confined to a wheelchair and has a significant head tilt, 15-diopter prism can be trialed to see whether it has a positive effect at correcting the head tilt. If successful, decrease the prism amount by 5 diopters and see whether it is still of benefit, and continue to decrease prism amount until no benefit is seen. Prescribe the smallest prism amount that still elicited a favorable response.

MIDLINE SHIFT EVALUATION

The visual midline shift syndrome is described by Dr. William Padula (Padula and Argyris 1996, 165) as an ambient visual dysfunction caused by neurological injury. Ambient visual process, also known as dorsal stream processing, provides information on spatial orientation, which is used for balance, movement, and coordination.

The examination is described as follows:

The patient is seated and instructions are as follows: "I am going to move this pen slowly across your field of view. I would like you to tell me when the pen is directly at the center of your nose. Please do not look at the pen, but try to focus straight ahead at a distance." You, sitting directly in front of the patient at approximately 2′ away, will start moving the pen from the left far periphery inward at a moderate pace. When the patient says "stop," you assess the location of the pen in relation to the patient's nose. You can repeat this test three times and estimate an average based on the patient's response. A consistent localization to the left or right is more reliable. If shift is found, trial of a 2–3 diopters yoked prism base toward the deviated side is suggested.

The theory is that the prism realigns the imbalance of the dorsal stream.

It is important to note not all gait and balance disorders are visual in nature. The visual system is simply one component to the balance system. Balance is comprised of three sensory inputs: vision, vestibular, and proprioceptive. Someone who has ototoxicity from gentamicin use is going to have balance difficulty arising from the vestibular input and someone with diabetic peripheral neuropathy is going to have balance difficulty due to the reduced sensory input coming from their feet.

TREATMENT FOR PHOTOSENSITIVITY

Photosensitivity can be very bothersome especially in the acute phase of the injury. Significant improvements can be made with prescribing tinted lenses. The best way to determine whether a tint will be helpful is by trialing several tints, such as blue, brown, gray, rose, blue blocker, and Anifra tint (12% blue-green). Often the best to use in an acute injury is the 15% blue tint.

HEMISPATIAL NEGLECT TESTING

Visual neglect (aka hemispatial neglect) is a condition that can occur after damage to one hemisphere of the brain. It most commonly occurs when the defect is in the right parietal lobe, and it usually leads to left neglect.

One method is performing confrontational visual fields. After determining that the patient can count fingers in each individual quadrant in the peripheral vision, present fingers on each hand, one in each hemifield, and determine whether the patient can count them all. If they consistently cannot, this is called the visual extinction phenomenon.

The next test is the clock drawing test. To perform this test, give the patient a sheet of paper with a large predrawn circle on it. Indicate the top of the page. Next, instruct the patient to draw numbers inside the circle and make the circle look like the face of a clock and then draw the hands of the clock to read "10 after 11." Table 5.1 explains the scoring for this test.

The last test that is used is the cancellation test. The subject is instructed to scan the document to locate all of a target letter, that is, J. In general, the

Table 5.1 Scoring for the Clock Drawing Test

Score	Description	Criterion
1	"Perfect"	No errors in the task
2	Minor visuospatial errors	a. Mildly impaired spacing of times b. Draws times outside circle c. Turns page while writing so that some numbers appear upside down d. Draws in lines (spokes) to orient spacing
3	Inaccurate representation of 10 after 11 when visuospatial organization is perfect or shows only minor deviations	a. Minute hand points to 10 b. Writes "10 after 11" c. Unable to make any denotation of time
4	Moderate visuospatial disorganization of times such that accurate denotation of 10 after 11 is impossible	a. Moderately poor spacing b. Omits numbers c. Perseveration: repeats circle or continues on past 12 to 13–15 d. Right–left reversal: numbers drawn counterclockwise e. Dysgraphia: unable to write numbers accurately
5	Severe level of disorganization as described in scoring of 4	See examples for scoring of 4
6	No reasonable representation of a clock	No attempt at all No semblance of a clock

Source: Data from Schulman, K., *Int. J. Geriatr. Psychiatry*, 8(6), 487, 1993.

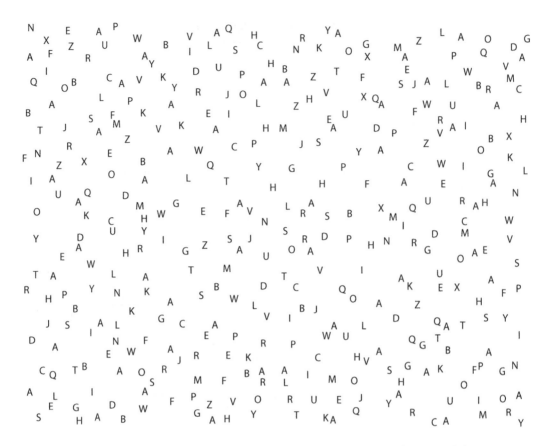

Figure 5.1 Example of letter cancellation task. (Reprinted with permission from Randel, J., Letter cancellation task, University of Kansas Medical Center, Kansas City, KS, November 2000, http://kumc. edu/, Web September 15, 2015.)

more cluttered the task, the more you are able to elicit the neglect. Please see Figure 5.1.

PERCEPTUAL EVALUATION

Visual perceptual evaluation is important to perform on patients with moderate-to-severe TBI, especially if a deficit is suspected. Chapter 9 reviews perceptual evaluation and treatment.

REFERENCES

Chen, J.W., Gombart, Z.J., Rogers, S., Gardiner, S.K., Cecil, S., and Bullock, R.M. 2011. Pupillary reactivity as an early indicator of increased intracranial pressure: The introduction of the neurological pupil index. *Surg Neurol Int.* 2:82. [Online.]

Padula, W.V. and Argyris, S. 1996. Post trauma vision syndrome and visual midline shift syndrome. *NeuroRehabilitation.* 6:165–171.

Randel, J., Letter cancellation task. Kansas City, KS: University of Kansas Medical Center, November 2000. http://kumc.edu/, Web September 15, 2015.

Schulman, K. 1993. Clock drawing and dementia in the community: A longitudinal study. *Int J Geriatr Psychiatry.* 8(6):487–496.

6

Ocular motility flow sheet and instructions

OCULAR MOTILITY

Fixation is worked on indirectly with pursuit and saccadic exercises by

1. Slowing down the exercise with pursuits
2. Having patient stay on target once they make a saccade

PURSUIT ACTIVITIES

1. Spoon pursuits
2. Fist passes
3. Pegboard rotator—inserting peg into board
4. Neurovision rehabilitator (NVR) visual-motor enhancer (VME) programs
5. Sanet vision integrator (SVI) rotator programs

SACCADE ACTIVITIES

Large angle/integrate peripheral awareness

1. Post-it saccades
2. Four-corner Hart chart saccades
3. NVR dynamic oculomotor processing (DOMP) programs
4. NVR ocular vestibular integrator (OVI) programs
5. SVI saccades: proactive/reactive programs
6. Wayne Saccadic Fixator
7. McDonald chart

Small angle/reading related

1. Michigan tracking (varying size font)
2. PS forms (lower level)

3. Hart chart
4. Percon saccades/saccadic workbook
5. CPT visual scan/visual search
6. Vogel track and read programs

Monocular versus binocular: Perform these activities monocularly, if the patient has any of the following:

1. Monocular amblyopia
2. Reduce acuity or reduce visual field of one eye
3. Presence of an eye turn
4. Decreased accommodation or convergence

SPOON PURSUITS

Purpose

To develop smooth pursuits and increase peripheral awareness

Equipment

- Glasses
- Eye patch
- Spoon

Duration

10 minutes

Set-up

Let the patient stand or sit erect with good posture.

Directions

1. Place an eye patch over one eye.
2. Let the patient hold the spoon with the convex side facing his or her eye with elbows slightly bent.

3. Let the patient fixate on the image of his or her face in the spoon.
4. Instruct the patient to move the spoon *slowly* in the following directions:
   a. Horizontal left and right
   b. Vertical up and down
   c. Oblique up and down
   d. Clockwise (CW)
   e. Counterclockwise (CCW)
5. Let the patient follow the spoon with their eye (without moving their head) while their arm moves the route smoothly and easily. Instruct the patient to continue to the point when they cannot see the image of their eye on the spoon. Let them try to feel their eyes moving.
6. Direct the patient to move only their arm and eyeball, making sure their head is not moving.
7. Repeat three times all of these directions.
8. Repeat for the other eye.

Variations

- As this activity is continued, let the patient increase their awareness of the other objects in the room without taking their spoon.
- Perform the procedure with each eye and, when successful, with both eyes.

NVR FIXATION ANOMALIES 1

Purpose

To enhance fixation anomalies (FAs)

Equipment

- NVR
- Hand remote
- Eye patch

Duration

5 minutes (each eye)

Set-up

- The patient should be 6′–8′ from the projection screen.
- Instruct the patient to stand up with good posture with feet shoulder width apart and hands relaxed at the sides.
- Let the patient hold the hand remote with the index finger of the preferred hand placed on the trigger.

Directions

1. Place the patch over the left eye.
2. Instruct patient to look at the screen and move their eyes slowly from left to right until they reach a cell with an underscore line.
3. Direct the patient to adjust the focus of their eyes so that the dots are as clear and stable as possible.
4. Direct the hand remote and place the remote's cursor on the first dot in the cell.
5. Once they feel that they are accurately aligned, they are to squeeze the trigger and shoot the dot.
6. Then, they are to immediately control fixation and keep the remote's cursor on the dot.
7. The goal is to keep the cursor steady on the dot for a period of time, which is set from the parameter option menu.
8. Each time that fixation is lost and the hand remote cursor comes off the dot, an auditory tone will sound, which is an alert.
9. Let the patient continue for the rest of the dots in the cell and then move to the next cell that is underscored.
10. When finished, move the patch over to the right eye.

Note

- The most important outcome is for the patient to be able to sustain fixation, and accurate auditory cue is very important as its feedback.
- It is important to stress to the patient that they must perform this task slowly and deliberately.

Variations

Add a balance board.

NVR FA 2

Purpose

To enhance FA

Equipment

- NVR
- Hand remote
- Eye patch

Duration

5 minutes (each eye)

Set-up

- The patient should be 6'–8' from the projection screen.
- Direct the patient to stand up with good posture with feet shoulder width apart and hands relaxed at the sides.
- Let the patient hold the hand remote with the index finger of the preferred hand placed on the trigger.

Directions

1. Patch the patient's left eye.
2. Direct the patient to start by shooting the central bull's-eye.
3. Instruct patient to relax and to feel their eyes, fixating the left dot on the first line in the first group on the left.
4. When the dot is steady and clear, they are to aim and place the hand remote's cursor on the dot and then squeeze the trigger and shoot the dot.
5. A correct response is reinforced by an auditory tone, while an incorrect one a different tone.
6. Once they successfully shoot the dot, they are to slowly trace the line with the hand remote's cursor until they reach the bottom dot.
7. Then, direct the patient to shoot that dot and continue to the next line or group.
8. Once patient has shot the last dot, they will shoot the number displayed on the bottom of the screen that corresponds to the number of the hatch lines they have shot.
9. Switch the patch to their right eye and repeat the process.

Note

- The most important outcome is for the patient to be able to sustain fixation and accurate visuomotor act as they trace the line; the auditory cue is very important as its feedback.
- It is important to stress to the patient that they must perform this task slowly and deliberately.

Variations

- You can adjust the separation of the lines by moving them closer to each other and making it harder by using the ± keys on the keyboard.
- Add a balance board.

NVR FA 3

Purpose

To enhance FA

Equipment

- NVR
- Hand remote

Duration

5 minutes (can be done monocularly or binocularly)

Set-up

- The patient should be 6'–8' from the projection screen.
- Instruct the patient to stand up with good posture with feet shoulder width apart and hands relaxed at the sides.
- Let the patient hold the hand remote with the index finger of the preferred hand placed on the trigger.

Directions

1. Instruct the patient to relax and feel their eyes and then look at the letter A at the top edge of the serpentine line and shoot it.
2. Next, they are to slowly trace the line with the hand remote cursor until they reach the cross-hatched lines.
3. When they reach the lines, they are to shoot the dot on the left side and then trace the line with the remote until they reach the dot on the right.
4. They must shoot the dot and then continue to the next line or group.
5. Once the patient has shot the last dot, they will follow the serpentine line to the letter B and shoot it.
6. They will shoot the number displayed on the bottom of the screen that corresponds to the number of the hatch lines they have shot.

Note

- Tell patient to visualize the serpentine line as a road they are going on and to always shoot the first dot on the left first.

Variations

- You can adjust the separation of the lines by moving them closer to each other and making it harder by using the ± keys on the keyboard.
- Add a balance board.

- Work on antisuppression by selecting red/blue and have the patient wear R/B glasses. Note that the images here are in grayscale; the NVR program that you have will be in color.

NVR VISUAL-MOTOR ENHANCER: PEGBOARD ROTATOR (FIGURE 6.1)

Purpose

To develop smooth pursuits. This activity is good for all patients.

Equipment

- Distance glasses
- NVR computer program
- Eye patch

Duration

10 minutes, two times each day

Set-up

1. Start by a monocular cover of one eye with the patch.
2. Let the patient stand about 10′ back centered in front of the large screen.
3. Log into the NVR program.
4. Select VME.
5. From the drop-down menu, select
   a. Speed 5–7 progress up to 12
   b. Targets 8
   c. Direction CW or CCW

d. Select both clockwise and counterclockwise and automatic (will automatically switch the letter that is highlighted)
e. Select which eye you will be training with

Directions

- Instruct the patient to use their eyes to guide their hand to track the letter that is blue.
- Let them be aware of the other letters on the board.
- When another letter turns blue, direct them to look at it first and then use their eyes to guide their hand to the letter, making sure that they are on it and will be able to shoot it out.
- Note that the beeping sound is the feedback to let them know they are off the target. They must make a correction to stop the sound. This is also true for the balance component.
- Repeat these steps with the other eye.

Variations

- Add a balance board.
- Add distractors.
- Add a metronome hold.
- Add a yoked prism.

DYNAMIC OCULOMOTOR PROCESSING 1 (FIGURE 6.2)

Purpose

To increase the speed of visual processing, especially for peripheral awareness, saccades, visually

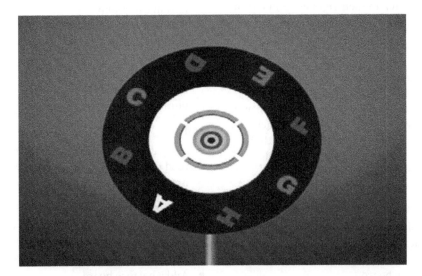

Figure 6.1 Visual-motor enhancer module. (Courtesy of Allen Cohen.)

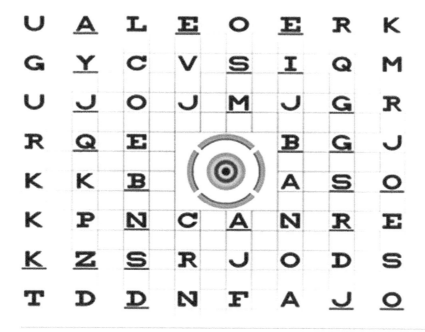

Figure 6.2 Dynamic ocular motor processing module. (Courtesy of Allen Cohen.)

guided graphomotor movements, and auditory, visual, and motor inputs, which are important for the vestibular ocular reflexes

Equipment

- Distance glasses
- NVR with hand remote
- Eye patch
- Prism
- Balance board

Duration

As required

Set-up

- Let the patient stand 8′–10′ centered in front of the screen.
- Ensure the patient is standing with good posture with feet shoulder width apart.
- Have the patient cover one eye.
- Log into the NVR program.
- Select DOMP 1.
- From the option menu, select
  a. First and last
  b. Targeted eye

Instructions

1. Encourage the patient to relax as this will help them expand their peripheral awareness of the entire chart.
2. Instruct the patient to move their eyes to the top left-hand corner of the screen.
3. Have the patient move the hand remote to the first letter and shoot it out.
4. Next, have the patient find the last letter of the first row with their peripheral vision first.
5. Next, direct the patient to move their eyes to the last target on the first line and then "visually guide" the hand shooter remote to the target and shoot it out.
6. Let the patient continue through the whole chart.

Note

If they shoot the wrong one, it will automatically go to the next.

Variations

- Select the second, and the second from the last, and the third, and the third from the last.
- Add a metronome.

- Add a prism monocularly to increase the sensory mismatch.
- Change the targets to the symbols in the target box on the parameter option menu.

HART CHART QUAD (FIGURE 6.3)

Purpose

To work on the accuracy of the large- and small-angle saccades

Equipment

- Hart chart and scissors
- Distance glasses
- Laser pointer (optional)

Duration

As required

Set-up

- Cut the Hart chart into four 5 × 5 squares.
- Place each 5 × 5 square approximately 3′ apart (forming four corners).
- Let the patient stand 4′–6′ from the chart.
- Ensure the patient is standing with good posture with feet shoulder width apart.

Instructions

1. Encourage the patient to relax as this will help them expand their peripheral awareness.
2. Instruct the patient to move their eyes to the top left square and read across the first line.
3. While keeping their eyes on the last letter of the first line, find the first letter of the chart to the right with their periphery vision; assure them this will not be clear.
4. Next, direct them to move their eyes smoothly and accurately to that letter and then read across the first line of that chart.
5. Repeat steps 3 through 4 for the chart directly below the current chart.
6. Go in CW order, and when the patient gets back to first chart, they will now read the second line and continue.
7. The goal is to finish the whole chart in CW and CCW order.

Note

- If they have trouble finding the first letter of the next chart with their peripheral vision, ask them to try to estimate where it would be or you can move the charts closer together.

Variations

- Add a balance board and also a metronome.

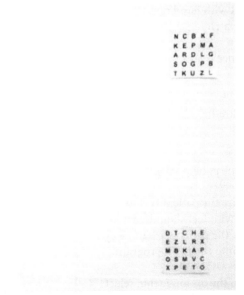

Figure 6.3 Hart chart quad.

FOUR-CORNER SACCADICS

Purpose

To help develop proper eye movement skills

Materials

• Laser light

Set-up

Let the patient patch their left eye, face a wall, and stand approximately 5′–10′ away.

Procedure

1. Instruct the patient to look to the upper-left corner. When direction is to "shift," let them move their eye to the upper right-hand corner of the room.
2. Tell them to try to move their eyes from the left corner to the right corner without moving their head.
3. On a command, let their eye shift to the lower right corner and then to the lower left corner.
4. After each fixation (at each corner), accurately aim a flashlight at each corner of the wall.
5. Repeat this procedure 10 cycles with two repetitions in CW and CCW direction.
6. Next, direct the patient to shift the patch to their right eye. Then repeat the procedure with their left eye.
7. When you can successfully perform this procedure with each eye, repeat these with both eyes open. Tell the patient to try to be aware of the objects in the room when shifting from corner to corner.
8. Repeat these while in balance and standing on a pillow.

Note

• If the patient cannot perform this activity without moving their head or body, instruct them to place a book or sponge on their head. If they move their head, the sponge or book should fall off. Tell them to try to perform this activity without allowing the book or sponge to fall off.
• The goal is to visualize the corner with their peripheral vision and then move their eye and accurately fixate the corner, followed by a visually guided movement of the laser light to accurately flash the corner.

MODIFIED HART CHART

Purpose

To help develop proper eye movement skills
To be used for patients with severe deficit of saccades

Materials

Hart chart and scissors

Set-up

• Cut the Hart chart into single vertical strips.
• Place two strips on a wall 2′ apart from each other.
• Let the patient stand (or sit) 4–5′ away.

Procedure

1. Follow the same instructions as those of Hart chart saccades. Let the patient call out the first letter on the left strip and then the first letter on the right strip.
2. Instruct the patient to move their eyes back to the first strip and call out the second letter on the left strip and then the second letter on the right strip.
3. Direct the patient to continue the step until they get into the last letter on each strip.
4. Let them try to feel their eyes move and try to make their eye movements smooth and accurate.

Variations

• Add another strip (three strips, 2′ apart).
• Add a metronome.
• Add a balance board.

WAYNE SACCADIC FIXATOR (FIGURE 6.4)

Purpose

To improve the quality of medium-angle saccades

Materials

• Wayne Saccadic Fixator

Set-up

• Have patient stand arm's length away from the instrument (eye level).

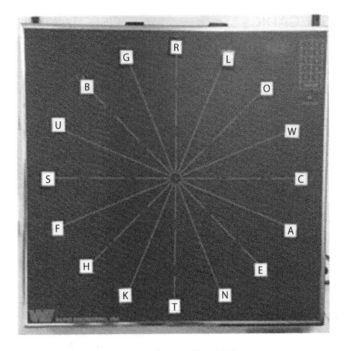

Figure 6.4 Wayne Saccadic Fixator. (Courtesy of Bernell.com.)

- Turn on the instrument with the dial located on the lower right side; this also controls the volume.
- Let the patient press 9, then 3, then enter, and then the red light to start.

Procedure

1. Instruct the patient to look at the center of the screen and be aware of their periphery.
2. Ask the patient to find the light with their peripheral vision.
3. Then, instruct the patient to bring their eyes to the light.
4. Then, direct them to push the light with their index finger.
5. Then, let them return their eyes back to the center and their hand back to their sides.
6. Repeat the process.

Variations

- Have the patient alternate hands.
- Work with visual memory.
- Add a balance board and also a metronome.

Availability: wayneengineering.com

SACCADIC WORKBOOKS (FIGURE 6.5)

Purpose

To improve small-angle saccades and also reading ability

Equipment

- Percon saccade packet

Set-up

- Have the patient seated.
- Place a packet on the table in front of the patient approximately 18″ away from the eyes.

Procedure

1. Have the patient read out loud underlined letters/numbers from top to bottom, left to right.

Note

- Can be timed
- Image source: www.bernell.com

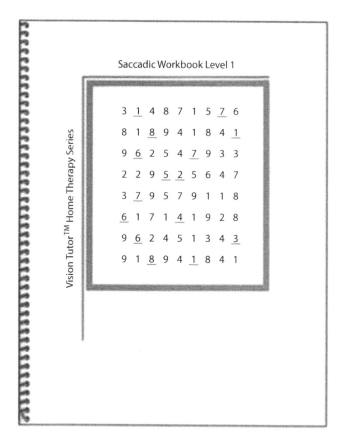

Figure 6.5 Saccadic workbook. (Courtesy of Bernell.com.)

NVR OVI (FIGURE 6.6)

Purpose

To increase peripheral awareness and saccades

Equipment

- Distance glasses
- NVR computer program
- Eye patch

Duration

As required

Set-up

- Start with a monocular cover of one eye with the patch.
- Instruct the patient to stand about 10′ back centered in front of the large screen.
- Log into the NVR program.
- Select OVI.

- From the drop-down menu, select
  - Cells—20
  - Weight—50
  - Vertical weight—50
  - Randomize
  - Cell distractor (when ready)
  - Voice assist
  - Targeted eye

Instructions

1. Instruct the patient to stand in front of the screen and look straight ahead at the bull's-eye and then shoot out the target.
2. Using their peripheral vision, locate the next lit target.
3. Direct the patient to bring their eyes to the target.
4. Let them use their eyes to guide their hand and shoot out the target.
5. Switch eye.

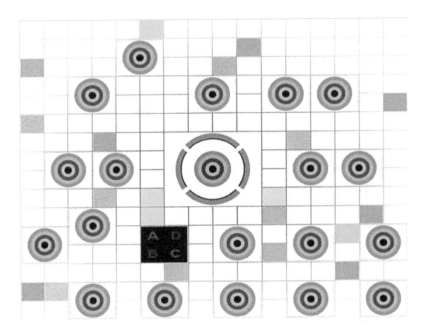

Figure 6.6 Ocular vestibular integrator. (Courtesy of Allen Cohen.)

Variations

- Add a metronome hold.
- OVI 2 balance.
- OVI 5 Stereo R/B glasses Can increase convergence or divergence.
- OVI 6 Add balance to OVI 5.

POST-IT SACCADES (FIGURE 6.7)

Purpose

To develop smooth and accurate eye fixations while increasing peripheral awareness

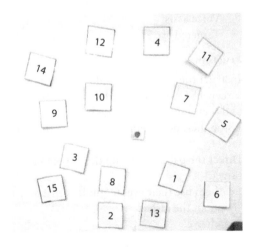

Figure 6.7 Post-it saccades.

Equipment

- Distance glasses
- 15 Post-it notes
- Laser light or flashlight
- Eye patch
- Tape
- Clear uncluttered wall or door space

Duration

10 minutes, two times each day

Set-up

- In the center of each Post-it note, instruct the patient to draw the numerals 1 through 15 about 2″ in height.
- On a piece of tape, let the patient make a circle "bull's-eye" (a circle sticker can be used).
- Direct the patient to place the "bull's-eye" on the wall at an eye level.
- Tell then the patient to randomly place the Post-its around the bull's-eye.

Directions

1. Instruct the patient to stand 6′ away from the wall, directly in front of the Post-its.
2. Direct them to place the eye patch over the right eye.

3. Let the patient to fixate on the "bull's-eye" and using their peripheral vision (side vision), tell them to be aware of the numbers around it.
4. (Using side vision) Let the patient locate number #1 Post-it and move their eye to it.
5. While fixating on the Post-it, instruct them to locate the "bull's-eye" and move their eye back.
6. Tell the patient to continue this through 2–15.
7. Repeat the process with the left eye.

Variations

- Take steps back if they can't see a number.
- Have someone call off the numbers in random order.
- Let the patient move closer to the wall as fixation improves (not closer than 4′).
- After you are proficient with this task, add a laser to light each card. The goal is to find the number with accurate eye movements and then accurately illuminate each card with a visually guided movement.
- Add a metronome.
- Let the patient perform these while standing on a pillow (*when prescribed*).

DOMP 2 AND DOMP 3 (FIGURE 6.2)

Purpose

To increase the speed of visual processing, especially for peripheral awareness, saccades, visually guided graphomotor movements, and auditory, visual, and motor inputs, which are important for the vestibular ocular reflexes

Equipment

- Distance glasses
- NVR with hand remote
- Eye patch
- Prism
- Balance board

Duration

As required

Set-up

- Instruct the patient to stand 8′–10′ centered in front of the screen.
- Ensure patient is standing with good posture with feet shoulder width apart.
- Have the patient cover one of their eyes.

- Log into the NVR program
- Select DOMP 2.

Instructions

1. Encourage the patient to relax as this will help them expand their peripheral awareness of the entire chart.
2. Instruct the patient to start by moving their eyes to the top left-hand corner of the screen.
3. Next, have the patient find (with their peripheral vision) the first letter that has an underscore.
4. Next, direct the patient move their eyes to the target.
5. Finally, let the patient "visually guide" the hand shooter remote to the target and shoot it out.
6. The patient then finds the next letter with an underscore with their peripheral vision.
7. Repeat steps 4 through 6 for the whole chart.

Note

If they shoot the wrong one, it will automatically go to the next.

Variations

- Add a metronome.
- Add a prism monocularly to increase the sensory mismatch.
- Change the targets to the symbols in the target box on the parameter menu.

VME 4 (FIGURE 6.1)

Purpose

To develop smooth pursuits with medium-angle saccades

Equipment

- NVR VME 4
- Hand remote

Set-up

- Same as VME 4
- Select starting speed at 5

Procedure

1. Have the patient shoot out the letter in blue and another letter will light up in either blue or red.

2. Instruct the patient to find the next letter with their peripheral vision.
3. Next, direct the patient to move their eyes to the letter.
4. Finally, let the patient move their hand remote to the blue or red letter and shoot it out.
5. Repeat the steps.
6. The goal is to attain 80% accuracy.

Note

- You can increase the speed.
- You can have the patient put on red/blue glasses to work on antisuppression.
- Add a balance board.
- Add a metronome.

COOPER'S BASIC SACCADES

Purpose

- To improve the accuracy and speed of fixation and small-/moderate-angle saccades

Equipment

- Reading glasses
- VTS3 computer program

Duration

As required

Set-up

- The patient should be seated in front of the computer screen 20" away.
- The patient should put the VTS3 glasses on over their reading glasses.

Directions

1. Let the patient sit at the table 16" from the screen.
2. Place the eye patch over the eye of the patient if working monocularly.
3. Ensure the patient is sitting up straight.
4. Log into the VTS3 program.
5. Select saccades.
6. Instruct the patient to look for an arrow placed on the screen and key into the joystick the orientation of the arrow.

Variations

- This can be performed monocularly or binocularly.

MICHIGAN TRACKING (FIGURE 6.8)

Purpose

- To improve the accuracy and speed of fixation and small-angle saccades
- To improve visual discrimination, left to right directionality, and eye movement skills required to read across a line

Equipment

- Glasses
- Pencil
- Eye patch
- Letter-tracking sheets
- Timer

Duration

10 minutes, two times each day

Set-up

- Let the patient sit at the table 16" from the paper.
- Place the eye patch over their eye if working monocularly.
- Ensure the patient is sitting up straight.
- Ensure proper lighting.

Directions

1. Each paragraph contains nonsense words. Let the patient know that their task is to find the letters of the alphabet and cross them off in order.
2. Instruct the patient to start the test by crossing out the first "A" they come across with on the line and then cross out the first letter "B," and so on, until they get to the letter "Z" at the end of the paragraph.
3. Direct them not to go backward to find the letter, but always go forward.
4. Tell them to continue until they have circled each letter of the alphabet in order.

Variations

- The patient can circle all of the same letters.
- They can do a word search such as finding the letters to spell "CAT."
- For speed/accuracy trade-off, record the time it takes to complete each paragraph.

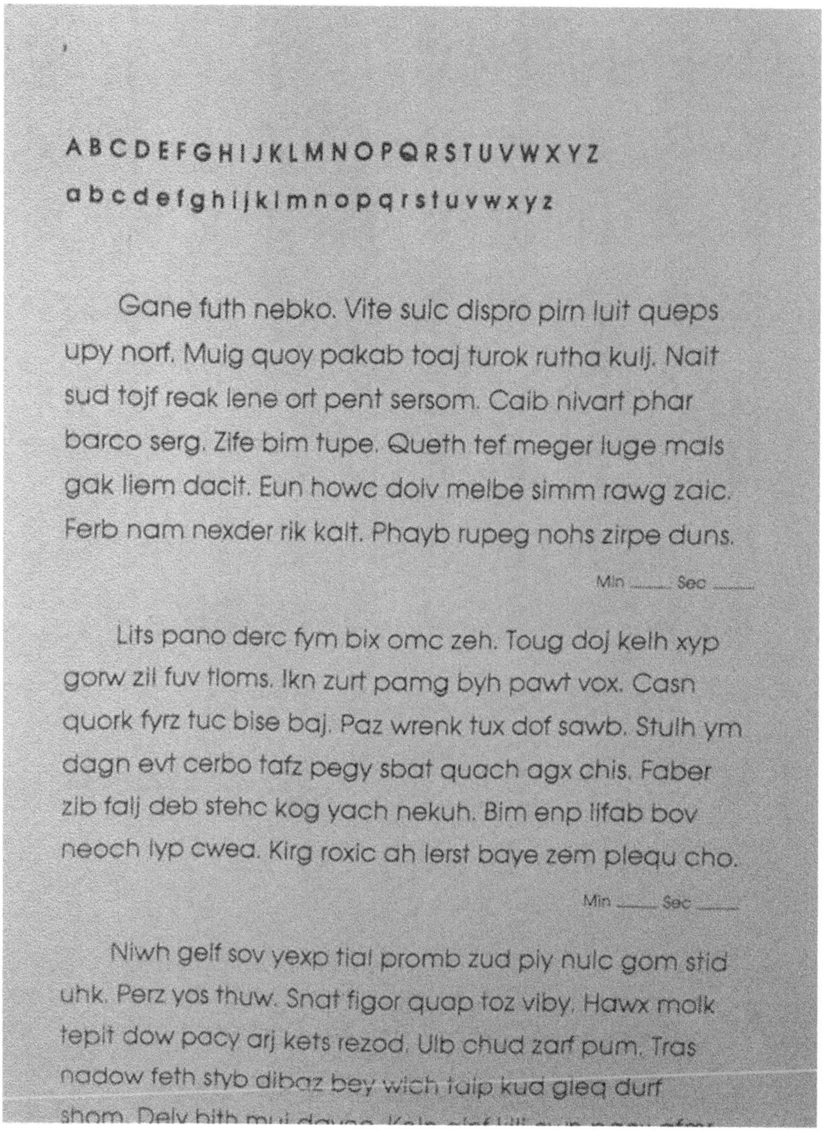
A B C D E F G H I J K L M N O P Q R S T U V W X Y Z
a b c d e f g h i j k l m n o p q r s t u v w x y z

Gane futh nebko. Vite sulc dispro pirn luit queps upy norf. Muig quoy pakab toaj turok rutha kulj. Nait sud tojf reak lene ort pent sersom. Caib nivart phar barco serg. Zife bim tupe. Queth tef meger luge mals gak liem dacit. Eun howc doiv melbe simm rawg zaic. Ferb nam nexder rik kalt. Phayb rupeg nohs zirpe duns.

Min ____ Sec ____

Lits pano derc fym bix omc zeh. Toug doj kelh xyp gorw zil fuv tloms. Ikn zurt pamg byh pawt vox. Casn quork fyrz tuc bise baj. Paz wrenk tux dof sawb. Stulh ym dagn evt cerbo tafz pegy sbat quach agx chis. Faber zib falj deb stehc kog yach nekuh. Bim enp lifab bov neoch lyp cwea. Kirg roxic ah lerst baye zem plequ cho.

Min ____ Sec ____

Niwh gelf sov yexp tial promb zud piy nulc gom stid uhk. Perz yos thuw. Snat figor quap toz viby. Hawx molk tepit dow pacy arj kets rezod. Ulb chud zarf pum. Tras nadow feth styb dibaz bey wich taip kud gleq durf

Figure 6.8 Michigan tracking.

HART CHART SACCADES (FIGURE 6.9)

Purpose

- To improve visual fixation skills, which are the most important aspects in reading

Goals

- To consistently call out the appropriate letter in order correctly
- To increase their speed and timing while learning to "see ahead" to the next section of the letters

Equipment

- Distance Hart chart
- Eye patch
- Clear uncluttered wall or door space

Duration

- 10 minutes, two times each day

Set-up

- Place a Hart chart on a uncluttered wall.
- Set a metronome time (when using).

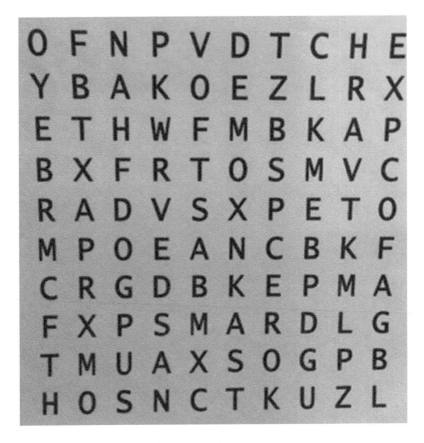

Figure 6.9 Hart chart.

Directions

1. Instruct the patient to call off the first letter on the first row and then the last letter of the first row.
2. Next, direct the patient to call off the first letter on the second row and then the last.
3. This will be called 1/10 since they are calling off letters in columns 1 and 10. Continue this procedure for the entire sheet.
4. If they are able to complete this exercise, then they should go back to the top of the chart and start calling off letters in columns 2 and 8, then 3 and 7, then 4 and 7.

Important Aspects

- Tell the patient to make sure that only their eyes are moving and not their head. Instruct the patient to perform this activity daily or as instructed using their glasses.

- When finding the letters, require them to attempt to visualize where the next letter is by expanding their peripheral awareness and then moving their eyes to the next letter.

Variations

- Perform these with a metronome waiting for the appropriate beats before finding the next letter.

Important Aspects

- Make sure only your eyes are moving and not your head. Perform this activity daily or as instructed using your glasses.
- When finding the letters, attempt to visualize where the next letter is by expanding your peripheral awareness and then move your eyes to the next letter.

```
O F N P V D T C H E
Y B A K O E Z L R X
E T H W F M B K A P
B X F R T O S M V C
R A D V S X P E T O
M P O E A N C B K F
C R G D B K E P M A
F X P S M A R D L G
T M U A X S O G P B
H O S N C T K U Z L
```

Figure 6.10 Example of Hart chart saccades, wherein the patient will read the first and last letters highlighted in the lighter color, then the second from the first, and the second from the last as highlighted in the darker color.

Variations

- Repeat these on a pillow when this modification is prescribed.
- Now, using a laser light, let the patient flash the fixated letter after they move their eye and fixate it. It is important that they first visualize where the letter is and then move their eye and fixate the letter and then visually guide their hand to accurately flash the letter.
- Let the patient perform these with a metronome waiting for the appropriate beats before finding the next letter (Figure 6.10).

SACCADIC WORKBOOK

Purpose

To improve small-angle saccades as well as reading ability

Equipment

- Saccade workbook

Set-up

- Have the patient seated.
- Place a packet on the table in front of the patient approximately 18″ away from their eyes.

Procedure

1. Have the patient read out loud the underlined letters/numbers from top to bottom, left to right.

Note

This can be timed.

COMPUTER VISUAL SCAN (FIGURE 6.11)

Purpose

- To improve the accuracy and speed of fixation and small-angle saccades
- To develop figure-ground

Equipment

- Distance glasses
- CPT computer program

Duration

As required

Set-up

- Let the patient sit at the table 16″ from the monitor with proper posture.

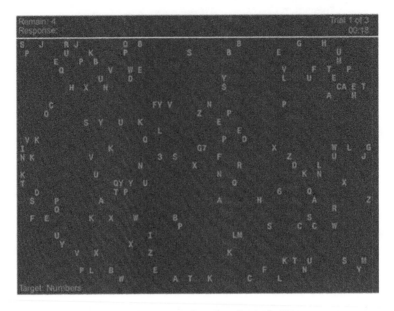

Figure 6.11 Computerized visual scan. (Courtesy of Rodney K. Bortel.)

- Instruct the patient to stand 10′ centered in front of the projector screen.
- Log into the CPT program.
- Select visual scan.
- From menu option, select
  - 20 symbols
  - 120 lowercase letters
  - 1 trial record

Directions

1. Instruct the patient to search for symbols in the array of lowercase letters. Let them do this as if they were reading a page. Tell them to start at the top and work their way left to right, top to bottom.
2. Direct them to use their eyes to find the symbol and then bring their mouse to it.
   a. Tell them to be aware of the whole page while they are completing the exercise.

Variations

- This can be monocular or binocular.
- This can be performed while sitting or standing with the projector.
- Add a metronome.
- Add a balance board.

COMPUTER VISUAL SEARCH (FIGURE 6.12)

Purpose

- To improve the accuracy and speed of fixation and small-angle saccades

Equipment

- Distance glasses
- CPT computer program

Duration

As required

Set-up

- Let the patient sit at the table 16″ from the monitor while ensuring proper posture.
- Log into the CPT program.
- Select visual search.
- From menu, select
  - Begin with three letters or numbers per sequence
  - Three rows
  - Three column

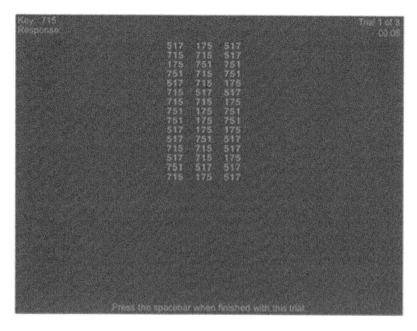

Figure 6.12 **(See color insert.)** Computerized visual search. (Courtesy of Rodney K. Bortel.)

- To increase the difficulty of this exercise, increase the number of rows and columns up to 5 × 10
- Lastly, increase the numbers in the sequence

Directions

1. Instruct the patient to look at the sequence on the top left-hand corner and to spend some time to picture it in their head.
2. Now, let them search for this exact sequence like they are reading a page, top to bottom, left to right.
3. Encourage patient not to look back at the sequence.
4. Document the following:
   a. Characters
   b. Rows
   c. Columns
   d. Time
   e. Errors

Variations

- This can be monocular or binocular.
- Add a metronome.
- Add a prism.

McDONALD CHART (FIGURE 6.13)

Purpose

- To increase the patient's peripheral awareness by becoming more aware of what is around them while they concentrate on the information straight ahead.
- To increase their central–peripheral flexibility, which will help their ability to organize visual information improve

Equipment

- Glasses
- Eye patch
- McDonald chart

Duration

10 minutes, two times each day

Set-up

- Cover one eye with the patch.
- Let the patient sit in a quiet place in a relaxed position with good posture.

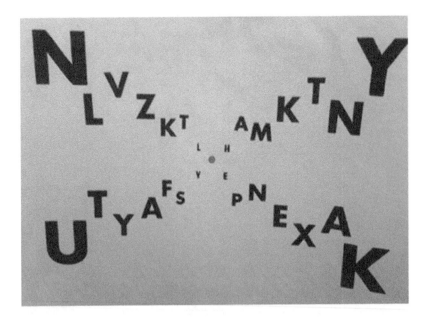

Figure 6.13 McDonald chart for peripheral awareness.

Directions

1. Instruct the patient to hold the chart at a distance of 13″ from their eyes.
2. Direct them to concentrate on the center dot.
3. While the patient is looking at the center dot, tell them be aware of the letters surrounding it without moving their eyes.
4. As they relax, require them to progressively pick up the symmetry of each set of four boxed letters as they increase in size.
5. Cover the other eye and repeat this exercise.

Important Aspects

- To maximize awareness of the patient's periphery, they have to "space out" or "phase through" the target a little bit.
- The more they relax, the more aware they will be of their periphery.

- At first, the patient may only be aware of the first letters immediately surrounding the dot. As they relax, they will progressively pick up the symmetry of each set of four "boxed" letters as they increase in size out to the edge.

Variations

- Repeat these on a pillow when this modification is prescribed.
- This may be done with plus lens to further open the patient's periphery.
- Let the patient tape record oneself when working alone, so they can concentrate at the task and then check the accuracy.
- Let them know that if they have trouble keeping their eye centered, they can cut a small hole in the middle and tape a small mirror behind it.

7

Accommodative flow sheet and therapy

ACCOMMODATION SET 1

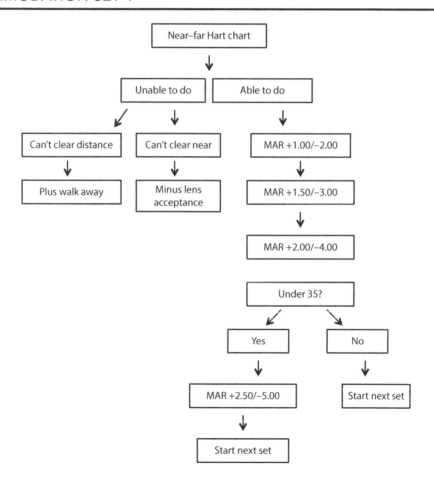

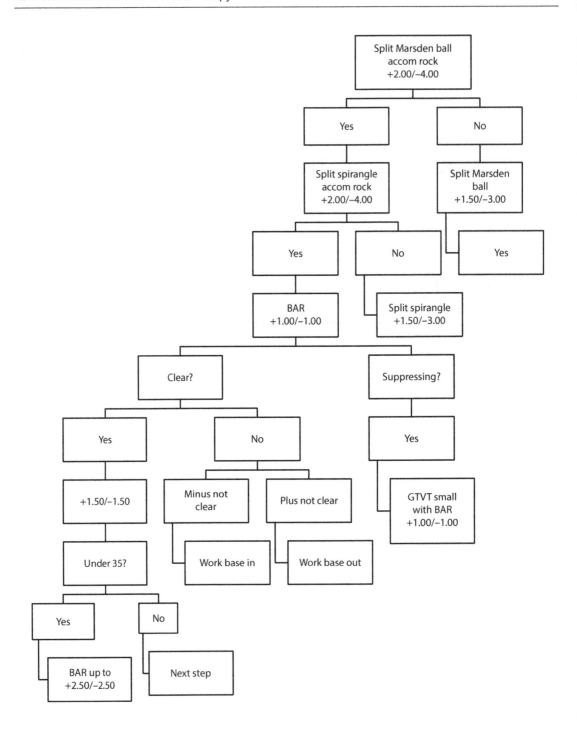

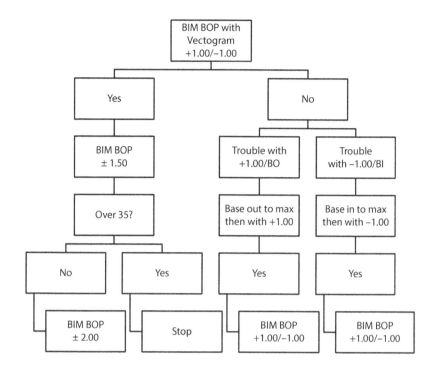

NEAR–FAR HART CHART (FIGURE 7.1)

Purpose

To develop flexibility in the change of focus when looking near to looking far

Equipment

- One large Hart alphabet chart
- One small Hart chart
- Eye patch

Duration

5 minutes for each eye

Set-up

- Tape a large chart to a wall, with a clear path to move backward.
- Instruct the patient to stand erect with good posture.
- Place the eye patch over the patient's eye.

Directions

1. Direct the patient to walk away from the large chart until the letters just start to blur, and then let them take one small step closer to the chart.

2. Hold the small letter chart 12″–16″ away from their eyes:
   a. Let the patient read the first line on the small chart all the way across.
   b. Instruct them to look up and read the second line on the large chart.
   c. Then, tell them to look down and read the third line on the small chart.
3. When the patient gets to the bottom of the chart, let them take one step back and see if they can still see the wall chart clearly: if so, repeat step 2; if not, record the distance traveled.
4. Switch the patch to the right eye and repeat steps 1 through 3.

Notes

- Tell the patient to wait until the letters are clear before reading it.
- Let them try to feel that their eyes change focus.

Variations

- This can be given as home exercise program (HEP) (5 minutes for each eye, twice a day)

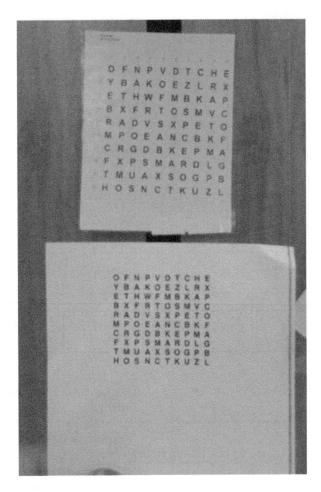

Figure 7.1 Near–far Hart chart.

- To increase difficulty, use the following:
  - Five letters far and then five letters near
  - Three letters far and then three letters near
  - Add a metronome, and clear each chart within three beats.

MINUS LENS ACCEPTANCE

Purpose

- To improve accommodative insufficiency (eye focusing)
- Starting point if patient cannot clear monocular accommodative rock (MAR) +1.00/−2.00 lens

Equipment

- Distance glasses (if applicable)
- −2.00 to −4.00 lens
- Eye patch
- Hart chart (should shrink letter size to 1/4th or use similar size chart)

Duration

4–5 repetitions

Set-up

- Instruct the patient to stand up with good posture ~10′ from the center in front of the Hart chart.
- Place the eye patch over their eye.

Directions

1. Direct the patient to hold the lens up to the uncovered eye and slowly walk forward to the chart until they find it difficult to read the first line on the chart. Stop.

2. Remove the lens and keep the chart clear.
3. Add lens back, read the third line on the chart and keep it clear.
4. Instruct the patient to walk ~1' forward and repeat adding lens and taking away.
5. Continue this process until they reach 2' in front of the chart and they can clear the lens.
6. Keep the chart clear.
7. Never use higher than −4.00 lens.
8. Ensure that the patient *does not* trombone the lens.

Note

• Instruct the patient to feel the eyes change focus.
• Once the patient can do this, try to use MAR +1.00/−2.00 again.

Variations

• This can be given as HEP.

MINUS LENS SORTING

Purpose

• To improve accommodative insufficiency (eye focusing) and detect small changes to accommodative demand
• Starting point if patient cannot clear MAR +1.00/−2.00 lens

Equipment

• Distance glasses (if applicable)
• Trial lenses (start with −0.50, then −0.50 increments, until −4.00)
• Eye patch
• Hart chart (should shrink letter size to 1/4th or use similar size chart)

Duration

4–5 repetitions

Set-up

• The patient should be seated holding small Hart chart 16″ away from the instrument.
• Place the eye patch over one eye.
• Trial lenses should be randomly scattered in front of the patient.

Directions

1. Instruct the patient that the goal of this activity is to place the lenses in order from the lens that causes the least amount of change in size of the Hart chart to the lens that minifies the letters the most.
2. The patient is to start by picking up any lens and hold it up to their eye. Let the patient try to clear the letters and at the same time tell them to be aware of any change in size the lens makes to the letters.
3. Direct the patient to put this lens down and take another one and do the same until all of the lenses are lined up from the most unchanged to the most changed. Let the patient double-check the results if necessary.
4. The therapist can look at the numbers printed on the lenses to see if the patient was accurate and record the result.
5. This test should be repeated for the other eye.

Note

• Instruct the patient to feel the eyes change focus
• Once patient can do this, try MAR +1.00/−2.00 again

SPLIT PUPIL ACCOMMODATIVE ROCK

Purpose

To improve accommodative insufficiency (eye focusing) and accommodative facility

Equipment

• Distance glasses (if applicable)
• Lens blank, start with −2.00 up to −5.00
• Eye patch
• Hart chart (use a 5 × 5 section of the large Hart chart)

Duration

2 repetitions per eye

Set-up

• Let the patient sit or stand 3'–4' away from the chart.
• Place the eye patch over one eye.

Directions

1. Instruct the patient to hold up the lens so the edge of the lens is halfway in their vision; the chart should now be double.

2. Make sure the lens is close to their eye, about ½″ away.
3. Direct the patient make the first line on the top chart clear and then read it; tell them to be aware that the lower chart is blurry.
4. Now clear the top line on the bottom chart and let the patient read it.
5. Tell the patient to continue this step going back and forth until they finish all the five lines.
6. Move the patch to the other eye and repeat the process.

Note

- Once the patient can clear the lens, we can increase the power.

Variations

- This can be given as HEP.

PLUS WALK AWAY

Purpose

- To help the patients who have trouble clearing the distance chart after reading the near chart
- To relax accommodative excess

Equipment

- Distance glasses (if applicable)
- Eye patch
- Low-power lens +0.50 to +1.00
- Hart chart

Duration

4–5 repetitions

Set-up

- Instruct the patient to stand with good posture ~2′ in front of the Hart chart.
- Place the eye patch over one eye.

Directions

1. Instruct the patient to hold the low-power lens up to the uncovered eye and read the first line on the chart and take lens away. Keep chart clear.
2. Remove lens and let the patient read the second line on the chart and then keep it clear.
3. Bring lens back to the uncovered eye and let the patient read the third line on the chart.
4. When the patient gets to the end of the chart, slowly back up and repeat steps 1 through 3.
5. Cue the patient to keep the chart clear.

6. Never use higher than a +1.00 lens.
7. Ensure the patient *does not* trombone the lens.
8. Continue until the patient can no longer clear the lens, which should be approximately 10′, less for the 1+ lens.

Notes

- The end point is hard to gauge and will not be the same for every patient; the point is to get them to relax their accommodation.
- Tell them to try to feel their eyes relax and be aware of the whole chart.
- As a hallway technique, this can be performed at distance and makes use of the expansive visual space of the hallway to promote accommodative relaxation.
- This can be given as HEP.

MONOCULAR ACCOMMODATIVE ROCK (FIGURE 7.2)

Purpose

To improve accommodative insufficiency and facility of each eye

Equipment

- Reading material or Michigan tracking 5p or 6p
- Plastic lens blanks
  - +1.00/−2.00 (as starting point)
  - +1.50/−3.00
  - +2.00/−4.00
  - +2.50/−4.50 (in patients under 30)
- Eye patch

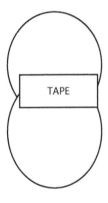

Figure 7.2 Example of how to tape plus and minus lens together to perform monocular accommodative rock.

Duration

3–5 minutes per eye

Set-up

- Occlude the patient's left eye.
- The reading material is held at 16″ (40 cm) away from the patient's eye or placed on a flat surface, which is also 16″ away from their eye.
- The patient is asked to hold lens set (taped together).

Procedure

1. The patient is asked to clear the print as they alternately hold the plus and then the minus lens in front of their right eye.
2. Give the patient as much time as necessary for them to clear and read the print, but ask the patient to try to decrease the time it takes to clear the lens.
3. The goal is to clear each lens within 1–2 seconds.
4. Repeat the procedure with the right eye occluded.
5. When the patient reach goal, go to the next set as shown in the "Equipment" section.

Notes

- If one eye is easier than the other, spend more time with the eye that has more difficulty.
- If the patient is experiencing difficulty at any level, suggest that patient try and get the "feeling" of looking close and crossing their eyes for the minus lenses or try and get the feeling of relaxing or staring for the plus lenses.
- Decrease the demand by moving page away until the print is clear and then moving back to 40 cm for the minus lenses or moving the card closer until the print clears and then move backing to 40 cm for the plus lenses.
- Decrease the demand by decreasing the power of the lenses for either plus or minus lens.
- This can be given for HEP.

SPLIT MARSDEN BALL (FIGURE 7.3)

Purpose

- To develop the speed/flexibility of eye focusing
- The step is between MAR and binocular accommodative facility (BAR)

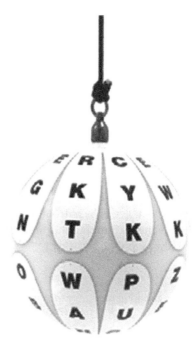

Figure 7.3 Marsden ball. (Courtesy of Bernell.com.)

This more challenging than MAR because this has to rapidly change focus from one eye to another.

Even though both eyes are open, the patient is not using both eyes at the same time.

Equipment

- Distance glasses (if applicable)
- One Marsden ball
- One prism (between 10 and 15 prism diopters)
- Trial lens (+2.00 in front of the right eye and −4.00 in front of the left eye)

Duration

5 minutes total

Set-up

- Hang Marsden ball at the patient's eye level.
- Have the patient stand 2′–3′ away from Marsden ball.
- Put trial lens on the patient.
- Have the patient hold the prism with the base facing down over the right eye.

Procedure

1. Tell patient about the following:
   a. You will see two balls, one on top of the other.

b. The top one is seen by your right eye and the bottom by your left eye.

c. Try to clear four letters of the top ball; you should feel your eyes relax focus.

d. Now move your eyes to the bottom ball.

e. Try to clear four letters of the bottom ball; you should feel your eyes increase focus.

2. Have the patient repeat steps a through e and try to decrease the time it takes for them to clear each ball.

3. Remove the trial lens from the patient's face and change the lens; +2.00 will be in front of left eye and −4.00 will be in front of right eye.

4. Repeat the instructions but this time c and e will be reversed.

Notes

- If patient cannot clear it, try moving them back 1′

- If they still cannot clear it, change the lens to +1.50/−3.00 (as also stated in the flow sheet).

- Image source: www.bernell.com

SPLIT SPIRANGLE (FIGURE 7.4)

Purpose

This is very similar to Marsden ball; the only differences that make it more challenging are

1. The letters are smaller
2. The working distance is shorter
3. Again even though both eyes are open, the patient is not using both eyes at the same time

Equipment

- Distance glasses (if applicable)
- Spirangle vectogram
- Vectogram holder
- Polarized glasses
- Trial lens (+2.00 in front of the right eye and −4.00 in front of the left eye)

Duration

5 minutes total

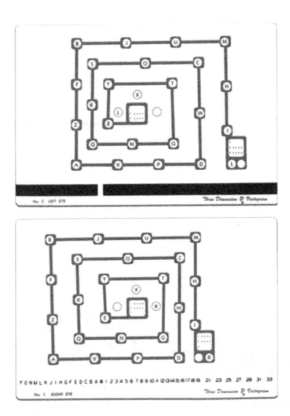

Figure 7.4 Spirangle vectogram. (Courtesy of Bernell.com.)

Set-up

- Place the spirangle vectogram with the R labeled on the top slot.
- Place the spirangle vectogram with the L labeled on the bottom slot.
- Have the patient sit 16″–18″ away from the vectogram.
- Put the trial lens on.
- Put the polarized glasses on.

Procedure

1. Tell the patient about the following:
   a. You will see spirangles, one on top of the other.
   b. The top one is seen by your right eye and the bottom by your left eye.
   c. Try to clear four large letters and one row of tiny letters of the top chart; you should feel your eyes relax focus.
   d. Now move your eyes to the bottom chart.
   e. Try to clear four large letters and one row of tiny letters of the bottom chart; you should feel your eyes increase focus.
2. Have the patient repeat steps a through e and try to decrease the time it takes for them to clear each chart.
3. Remove the trial lens from the patient's face and change the lens; +2.00 will be in front of the left eye and −4.00 will be in front of the right eye.
4. Repeat these instructions but now c and e will be reversed.

Note

- If the patient cannot see it clearly, change lens to +1.50/−3.00.
- Image source: www.bernell.com

BINOCULAR ACCOMMODATIVE FACILITY (FIGURE 7.5)

Purpose

To develop the speed/flexibility of eye focusing when both eyes are working together (this is the first activity that requires binocular vision)

Equipment

- Distance glasses (if applicable)
- Flip lenses
  - ±1.00 (as starting point)
  - ±1.25, ±1.50, and ±1.75
  - ±2.00, ±2.50 (for patients under 35)
- Reading material or MT 5p or 6p
- Red/green (or polarized) bar reader
- R/G (or polarized) glasses

Duration

5 minutes total

Set-up

- The polarized or R/G bar reader is placed on the reading material or MT5p/6p.
- The patient should wear polarized or R/G glasses.
- Have the patient sit 16″–18″ away from the reading material.

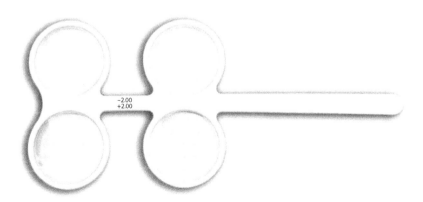

Figure 7.5 Accommodative flipper: accommodative flipper. (Courtesy of Bernell.com.)

Procedures

1. Flip lenses (±1.00) are held before the patient's eyes and the patient is instructed to clear the print.
2. The patient reads one line of letters and the flip lenses are flipped to the other side.
3. The patient is asked to clear and read the next line.
4. The therapist emphasizes that the reading material should always be visible through the stripes of the Polaroid or R/G material.
5. The patient should feel their eyes "focus" with the −1.00 lens and "relax" with the +1.00 lens.
6. The patient should clear each side within 1–2 seconds and try to decrease the time it takes for them to clear each side.
7. When the goal is reached, go to the next set as shown in the "Equipment" section.

Notes

- This can be given for HEP.
- This is when things start to get a bit complicated because the patient is binocular (using two eyes together), and therefore, if the patient has binocular problems, this will manifest during this activity, thus making it challenging.
- Try to follow the flow sheet for guidance when the patient is suppressing or had trouble clearing one side.
- Here is the general guideline:
  - In suppressing, work on antisuppression at near (i.e., GTVT).
  - If the patient cannot clear minus or words become double with minus lens: work base-in ranges at near
  - If the patient cannot clear plus or words become double with plus lens: work base-out ranges at near

GTVT WITH FLIP LENS (FIGURE 7.6)

Purpose

To add antisuppression and binocular alignment for patients that are suppressing on BAR

Equipment

- Distance glasses (if applicable)
- Small GTVT chart
- R/G glasses: Flip lenses (start with ±1.00)

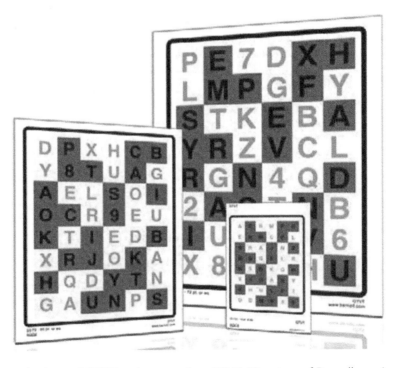

Figure 7.6 **(See color insert.)** GTVT antisuppression: GTVT. (Courtesy of Bernell.com.)

Duration

5 minutes total

Set-up

- Place small GTVT chart at the patient's eye level.
- Have the patient stand or seated 16″ away from the chart.
- Let the patient wear R/G glasses.

Procedures

1. Flip lenses (±1.00) are held before the patient's eyes and the patient is instructed to
   a. See all the letters on the first line
   b. Clear and read the letters on the first line
   c. Make sure the letters are aligned
   d. Flip the lens and repeat steps a through c for the second line
2. Continue steps a through d for the whole chart.
3. The goal is to clear each side within 1–2 seconds, to not suppress, and to have the letters aligned.
4. When the goal is reached, try to go back to regular BAR.

Notes

- The main goal is to not suppress.
- Not as concerned if the letters are drifting; will work on that with other activity (BIM/BOP), although it tells you the patient needs to work on binocularity.
- When the patient tries to clear +1.00 and the letters drift, tell them to try to feel their eyes cross and get them aligned.
- If the patient tries to clear −1.00 and the letters drift, tell them to try to feel their eyes relax and take a deep breath.
- This can be given for HEP.
- Image source: www.bernell.com.

BASE-IN MINUS, BASE-OUT PLUS (BIM BOP) (FIGURE 7.7)

Purpose

(For the last step) To train the eye to converge or diverge independent of eye focusing

Equipment

- Distance glasses (if applicable)
- Clown vectogram
- Spirangle vectogram
- Vectogram holder
- Polarized glasses
- Flip lenses
  - ±1.00 (starting point)
  - ±1.25, ±1.50, and ±1.75
  - ±2.00, ±2.50 (for patients under 35)

Duration

5 minutes total

Set-up

- Place the whole clown vectogram on the top slot.
- Place the whole spirangle vectogram on the bottom slot.
- Have patient sit 16″–18″ away from the vectogram.
- Put polarized glasses on.

Procedure

1. Flip lenses (+1.00) are held before the patient's eyes and the patient is instructed to look at the spirangle.
2. The therapist will slowly move the spirangle vectogram to position 3.
3. Ask the patient if they are able see the spirangle as 3D and able to keep it clear and single.
4. Have the patient flip lens over −1.00 and the patient is instructed to look at the clown.
5. The therapist will slowly move the clown vectogram to C.
6. Ask the patient if they are able to keep the clown 3D, clear, and single.
7. Have the patient flip the lens over +1.00 and look back at the spirangle and get it clear and single.
8. The therapist will slowly move the spirangle to 5.
9. Repeat steps 3 through 8:
   a. Increasing clown vectogram from C to E to G to I, etc.
   b. Increasing spirangle vectogram from 3 to 5 to 7 to 9, etc.
10. The goal is to get to the clown vectogram K spirangle 18.
11. When the goal is reached, go to the next flip lens as described in the "Equipment" section.

Notes

- Have the patient use a pointer to localize letters with the spirangle.

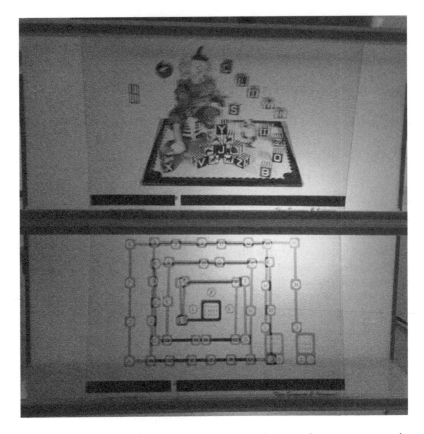

Figure 7.7 Set-up for BIM BOP, clown vectogram on top, and spirangle vectogram on bottom.

- Have the patient to decrease time it takes to get vectogram to be clear and single with every flip.
- If the patient has difficulty with +1.00 and spirangle, work on the spirangle and +1.00 only, and then reintroduce the clown and −1.00 (also see the modified BIM BOP).
- If patient has difficulty with −1.00 and clown vectogram, work on the spirangle and −1.00 only, and then reintroduce the spirangle and +1.00 (also see the modified BIM BOP).

MODIFIED BIM BOP

Purpose

To be used if the patient has trouble with one vectogram/lens in particular

Equipment

- Same as BIM BOP but only need the vectogram and the corresponding flipper that is challenging (for base in, it would be minus lens; for base out, it would be plus lens)

Duration

5 minutes total

Set-up

- Same as BIM BOP but just the vectogram and the side of the flipper that is challenging

Procedure

For ±1.00/Spirangle

1. Slowly slide the spirangle from zero position all the way out, while asking the patient to keep it single and 3D stop when it becomes double.
2. Go back three steps (i.e., if it became double at 10, go back to 7).
3. Ask the patient to keep it single.
4. Place +1.00 flip lens over the patient's eyes and ask them to keep the spirangle one.
5. Now slowly slide the spirangle further out until it becomes double.
6. Keep on pushing the patient to keep spirangle single and clear while you increase the

demand; if they cannot do it, take away the +1.00 lens and introduce it again when you think they are making progress.

For −1.00/Clown vectogram

1. Slowly slide the clown from the zero position all the way out, while asking the patient to keep it single and 3D stop when it becomes double.
2. Go back three steps (i.e., if it became double at H, go back to F).
3. Ask the patient to keep it single.
4. Place −1.00 flip lens over the patient's eyes and ask them to keep the clown one.
5. Now slowly slide the clown further out until it becomes double.
6. Keep on pushing the patient to keep the clown single and clear while you increase the demand; if they cannot do it, take away the −1.00 lens and introduce it again when you think they are making progress.

Note

It will be helpful to understand the following:

- With base in (clown vectogram), the patient's eyes have to diverge or relax; when they have to look through a −1.00 lens, the patient has to increase their accommodation, which naturally brings the eyes closer in (converge) so the patient has to actively diverge (or move their eyes apart) even more in order to keep the clown single.
- With the base out (spirangle), the patient's eyes have to cross (converge); when the patient uses a +1.00 lens, the patient has to relax their accommodation, which naturally brings the eyes out (or diverge) so the patient has to actively converge even more in order to keep the spirangle single.

8

Binocular section

Convergence insufficiency

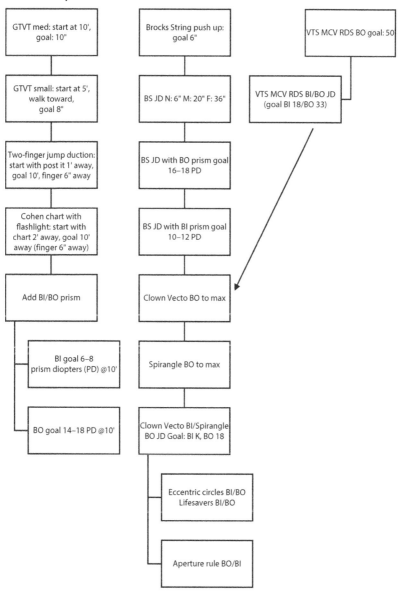

GTVT med: start at 10', goal: 10"

GTVT small: start at 5', walk toward, goal 8"

Two-finger jump duction: start with post it 1' away, goal 10', finger 6" away

Cohen chart with flashlight: start with chart 2' away, goal 10' away (finger 6" away)

Add BI/BO prism

BI goal 6–8 prism diopters (PD) @10'

BO goal 14–18 PD @10'

Brocks String push up: goal 6"

BS JD N: 6" M: 20" F: 36"

BS JD with BO prism goal 16–18 PD

BS JD with BI prism goal 10–12 PD

Clown Vecto BO to max

Spirangle BO to max

Clown Vecto BI/Spirangle BO JD Goal: BI K, BO 18

Eccentric circles BI/BO Lifesavers BI/BO

Aperture rule BO/BI

VTS MCV RDS BO goal: 50

VTS MCV RDS BI/BO JD (goal BI 18/BO 33)

Convergence excess

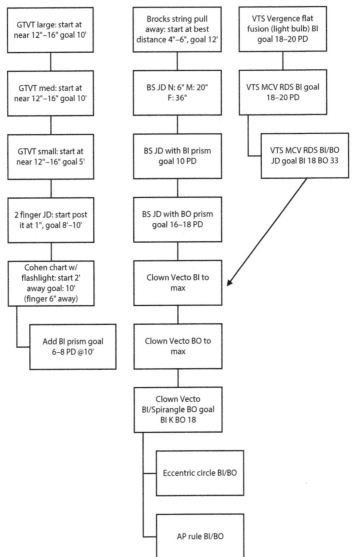

ANOTHER MORE GENERAL FLOW

Esophoria (convergence excess)

Phase 1

1. McDonald chart
2. Brock's string: start at a close range, where it is easy for the patient to converge accurately on the ball, then three bead jump
3. GTVT medium
4. Multiple-choice vergence (MCV; VTS) (base in [BI])
5. Two-finger jump duction

Phase 2

1. MCV jump ductions (BI and base out [BO])
2. Clown vectogram (BI)
3. Cohen chart with BI prism
4. GTVT small with BI prism (Tables 8.1 through 8.3)

Phase 3

1. BIM/BOP (±1.00 up to ±2.00) with a clown vectogram/spirangle vectogram
2. Aperture rule (BI; double aperture)
3. Lifesavers/eccentric circles (BI)

Table 8.1 Accommodation for >35 years old or patients that are having difficulty

Activity	Goal	Date completed
Near–far Hart chart	Far chart at 15′ away Near chart 10″ from the eye	
Minus lens sorting	Sort from −0.50 to −4.00 accurately with 0.25 increments	
Split pupil accommodation rock	Rock between plano and −3.00 lens	
Minus lens tromboning	With near Hart chart 16″ from the eye, clear up to −3.00 lens	
BAR ±0.75 up to ±1.50 with suppression check	Clear within 1–2 seconds each side without suppression	

Table 8.2 Convergence for >35 years old or patients that are having difficulty

Activity	Goal	Date completed
Polarized fusion sheet	To align the targets at 10″ away from each other with 20 BO prism	
Barrel card	To fuse all three barrels with the card touching the nose	
Pointer in the straw	To put the pointer in the straw accurately 10 times with the straw 4″ away from the nose	

Table 8.3 Divergence for >35 years old or patients that are having difficulty

Activity	Goal	Date completed
Brock's string push away	To converge accurately from 1″ to 5′	
Brock's string jump ductions	To see a single bead at 4″, 20″, and 4′ with 7 PD BI prism	
Polarized fusion sheet	To align targets at 16″ away from each other with 14 PD BI prism	
Quoits vectogram standing with localization	To be able to maximize out BI at 16″ away from the chart	

Note: Add +1.00 flipper to all divergence activities if they are not wearing their reading glasses.

Exophoria (convergence insufficiency)

Phase 1

1. Brock's string
2. Two-finger jump duction
3. Pointer in the straw
4. Computer MCV (BO)
5. Clown vectogram (BO with localization)

Phase 2

1. Spirangle (BO with localization)
2. Dynamic reader with BO prism
3. GTVT with BO prism

Phase 3

1. Aperture rule (BO; single aperture)
2. BIM/BOP (±1.00 up to ±2.00) with a clown vectogram/spirangle vectogram
3. Lifesavers/eccentric circles (BO)

HOME THERAPY

Convergence insufficiency

1. Two-finger jump duction
2. Brock's string push up and Brock's string jump ductions

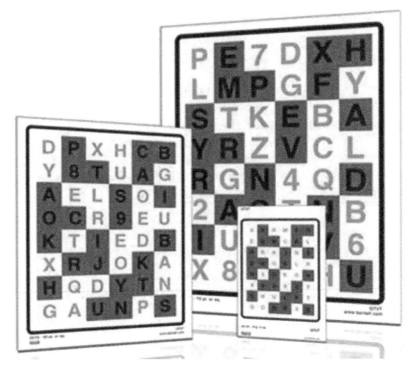

Figure 8.1 GTVT. (Reprinted with permission from Bernell.com.)

3. GTVT medium
4. Pointer in the straw
5. Barrel card
6. Fusion faces
7. Eccentric circles/lifesaver cards (opaque)*

Convergence excess

1. Two-finger jump duction
2. McDonald chart
3. Brock's string pull away, Brock's string jump ductions
4. GTVT medium
5. Eccentric circles/lifesaver cards (clear)†

GTVT (FIGURE 8.1)

Purpose

To decrease suppression and improve binocularity

* For activities that they can do base out and base in, they need to do base out first, get good at it, and then go do base in.

† For activities that they can do base out and base in, they need to do base out first, get good at it, and then go do base in.

Equipment

- GTVT chart (small, medium, or large)
- R/G glasses

Set-up

- Place the GTVT chart at the eye level.
- Have the patient stand at a proper distance.

Procedure

1. Have the patient look at the chart without R/G glasses.
2. Tell patient that if their eyes are working together, they should see all the letters the way they look now, evenly spaced apart.
3. Have the patient put R/G glasses on and ask them to describe what they see.
   a. If the light-colored letters disappear and the red lens is on their right eye, then they are suppressing their left eye, and vice versa; they should try to blink their eyes several times to break the suppression.
   b. If the letters are crossing, then their eyes are drifting outward and therefore they need to cross their eyes to align them.

c. If the letters are separating outward, then their eyes are drifting inward and therefore they need to relax their eyes to align them.

4. Once they are not suppressing and have the letters relatively aligned, they should move closer or further from the chart depending on the flow sheet.

Notes

- If the patient is suppressing or cannot get the letters to align, they can have them move closer or further away from the chart to a point where they can achieve it and start from there.
- It is okay if the patient cannot see all the letters on the chart at the same time, as long as they can see all the letters on the row they are looking at.

TWO-FINGER JUMP DUCTION

Purpose

To teach the two eyes to aim at a target and accurately jump their eyes from one distance to another

Equipment

Post-it sheet with a letter printed on it

Set-up

- Place a Post-it with a letter on the wall eye level.
- Instruct the patient to stand erect and balanced 1′ away from the wall.

Instructions

1. Instruct the patient to hold their index finger up at the nose level about 6″–8″, from their face.
2. Direct the patient to look at the letter on the Post-it: Let them feel their eyes focus the letter and fuse the image into a single image. Tell the patient that while they are focused on this letter, let them be aware of their finger that they are holding up and be aware that it has a ghost image next to it.
3. The goal is to maintain this experience (one fused letter on the Post-it and two fingers) for 5 seconds.
4. Then instruct the patient again to slowly aim their eyes to look at their raised finger.

Now, their goal is to fuse the two images of their finger into one. Tell them to be aware of the letter on the Post-it, which should appear to be double now.

5. Their goal is to maintain this experience for 5 seconds.
6. Then direct the patient to jump their eyes to the Post-it and repeat the cycle.
7. Their goal is to perform 10 jumps and 3 repetitions with a 1 minute rest between repetitions.
8. Next, direct the patient to step 1′ back from the Post-it and repeat the process.

Note

- If they cannot see the two Post-its when looking at their finger, have them blink their eyes or flash a light on the Post-it note.

COHEN CHART (FIGURE 8.2)

Purpose

To decrease suppression and improve binocularity

Equipment

- Cohen chart
- R/G glasses
- Prism bar

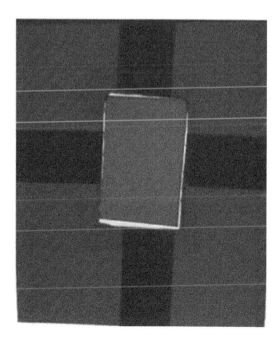

Figure 8.2 **(See color insert.)** Cohen chart. (Created by Allen Cohen.)

Set-up

- Place the Cohen chart at the eye level.
- Let the patient stand 2′ away from the chart.

Procedure

1. Ask the patient to first look at chart without R/G glasses; tell them, "if your two eyes are working together, this is what you should see, a black cross and a red box through the middle."
2. Then have the patient put on R/G glasses and ask them what they see.
   a. If they only see the black cross or the red box, they are suppressing one eye and they should try to blink and see if they can see them both at the same time.
   b. If the red box is skewed to the left (the red lens is in front of the right eye), then their eyes are underconverged and they should try to cross their eyes to get it to the center.
   c. If the red box is skewed to the right, then their eyes are overconverged and they should try to take a deep breath and relax to try to get it centered.
3. Once they are able to maintain the view for 5 seconds, have them move 1′ back and repeat the cycle.

4. Once they are able to get 10′ away, you can now introduce the prism (BI or BO depending on their disorder) in front of either eyes and again have them align the image.

Variation

Use a Cohen chart with two-finger jump duction: Have them hold up their index finger 6″–8″ away from their eyes (aligned with their nose), and while they are looking at the chart, make sure they see two fingers, and when they move their eyes behind their finger, they should see two charts: one red and one green. If they cannot see them, make them move closer till they can, and then let them try to step backward; the goal is 10′ distance.

BROCK'S STRING PUSH UP (FIGURE 8.3)

Purpose

To develop the ability of the two eyes to aim at the same point and converge/cross (for people who have convergence insufficiency)

Equipment

- 4′–6′ of string with one bead

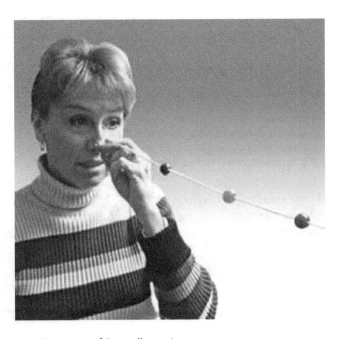

Figure 8.3 Brock's string. (Courtesy of Bernell.com.)

Set-up

- Instruct the patient to fasten one end of the string to any convenient object at or slightly below the eye level.
- Make the patient hold the other end of the string between their thumb and forefinger, just below the bridge of their nose.
- Let the patient place one bead 12″ away from their nose and push the rest (which are not needed for this activity) all the way back.

Procedure

1. Direct the patient to look at the bead. They should see one bead and two strings emerging from the sides of their face and meeting at the bead forming a "V." This is the normal response.
2. Let the patient slowly bring the bead closer and fixate on the bead. Tell them to feel their eyes aimed at the bead, keeping the bead clear and single with two strings crossing at the bead.
3. Their goal is to bring the bead up to 2″–3″ from their nose, seeing one bead and two strings aimed at the bead.
4. Instruct the patient that if at any time the bead doubles or if the strings cross in front or behind the bead, stop and aim their eyes until they are able to refocus. If this is not possible, tell them to slowly bring the bead away from them until they are able to focus the bead and then start bringing it toward them again.

Notes

- Perform the procedure with the patient standing and in balanced.
- Use the lenses prescribed by the doctor.
- While they are focusing on a specific bead, tell them to be aware of their peripheral vision.
- While they are focusing on a bead or shifting their eye between beads, let them try to be aware of how their eyes feel.
- If the string crosses in front of the bead (they are looking at), tell the patient that their eyes are overconverged and they need to take a deep breath and relax to bring the cross closer to the bead.
- If the string crosses behind the bead (they are looking at), tell the patient that their eyes are underconvergence and they need to strain/make their eyes cross in order to bring the cross closer to the bead.

BROCK'S STRING PULL AWAY

Purpose

To develop the ability of the two eyes to aim at the same point and diverge/uncross (for people who are convergence excess)

Equipment

- 4′–6′ of string with one bead

Set-up

- Instruct the patient to fasten one end of the string to any convenient object at or slightly below the eye level.
- Make the patient hold the other end of the string between their thumb and forefinger, just below the bridge of their nose.
- Let the patient place one bead 6″–8″ away from their nose and push the rest (which is not needed for this activity) all the way back.

Procedure

1. Direct the patient to look at the bead. They should see one bead and two strings emerging from the sides of their face and meeting at the bead forming a "V." This is the normal response.
2. Instruct the patient to slowly bring the bead further away from their nose and fixate on the bead. Let them feel their eyes aimed at the bead, keeping the bead clear and single with two strings crossing at the bead.
3. Their goal is to bring the bead up to 12″ away from their nose, seeing one bead and two strings aimed at the bead.
4. If at any time the bead doubles or if the strings cross in front or behind the bead, instruct the patient to stop and aim their eyes until they are able to refocus. If this is not possible, tell them to slowly bring the bead away from them until they are able to focus the bead and then start bringing it toward them again.

Notes

- Perform the procedure with the patient standing and in balanced.
- Use the lenses prescribed by the doctor.
- While they are focusing on a specific bead, tell them to be aware of their peripheral vision.

- While they are focusing on a bead or shifting their eye between beads, let them try to be aware of how their eyes feel.
- If the string crosses in front of the bead (they are looking at), tell them that their eyes are overconverged and they need to take a deep breath and relax to bring the cross closer to the bead.
- If the string crosses behind the bead (they are looking at), tell them that their eyes are underconverged and they need to strain/make their eyes cross in order to bring the cross closer to the bead.

BROCK'S STRING JUMP DUCTIONS

Purpose

To develop the ability of the two eyes to aim at the same point. It further develops the patient's ability to shift their eyes in a coordinated fashion from one point in space to another point quickly and easily without suppressing (turning off) the information of one of their eyes.

Equipment

- 4'–6' of string with three beads of different colors. The beads are spaced along the string.

Set-up

- Instruct the patient to fasten one end of the string to any convenient object at or slightly below the eye level.
- Make the patient hold the other end of the string between their thumb and forefinger, just below the bridge of their nose.

Procedure

1. Direct the patient to look at the far end of the string. They should see one marble and two strings emerging from the sides of their face and meeting at the far bead forming a "V." This is the normal response.
2. The near beads should now appear doubled, and both strings should be at the same height. If they see one string, they are suppressing one eye (the right eye sees the left string, while the left eye sees the right string). If this occurs, make the patient blink their eyes rapidly.
3. Next, instruct the patient to shift both eyes to the nearer bead. It should be clear and single with both strings meeting at it and forming an

"X." The far bead should appear double. The goal is to perform 10 jumps with 1 minute rest and then repeat the procedure three times.

4. If the patient can perform the aforementioned exercise successfully and accurately, sustaining the V or X, direct the patient to move the closest bead 1″ nearer to their face and the furthest bead 1″ further away from their face. The middle bead does not need to move.
5. Have the patient shift their eye from one bead to another. The "X" should immediately be seen with the center of the "X" exactly at the bead.
6. Let the patient shift back to the farthest bead and see the "V."
7. The goal is to converge their eyes and look at a bead placed 2″–3″ from their nose. They should see it single and clear with the awareness of other beads being double along the string.

Notes

- Same notes as pull away and push up.
- Use the lenses prescribed by the doctor (if the patient is older than 45 and has bifocals, they need to use top of bifocal to view far and middle bead and bottom of bifocal to view near bead).
- It is important to make smooth controlled jumps, i.e., when jumping from near to middle bead.

Variation

- Add a BI prism for esophoria (convergence excess) up to ~12 PD BI for near distances and ~9 PD for far distances.
- Add a BO prism for exophoria (convergence insufficiency) up to ~16 PD at all distances.

VTS3 VERGENCE/MULTIPLE-CHOICE VERGENCE

Purpose

To work on vergence range (improve binocular dysfunction, CI, CE): computerized

Equipment

- VTS3 Software
- LCD goggles and game controller

Set-up

- Have the patient seated approximately 18″ away from computer monitor at the eye level.
- Double click of VTS3, and click the "monitor" option.

- Make sure to confirm that the right eye sees "R" and the left eye sees "L"; click "this view is correct" and click next.
- Type in the patient information.
- Have the patient put on the goggles and hold on to the remote.

Procedure for MCV majority of patients

For convergence insufficiency: Select "RDS" and "medium" size; then select "BO," keep rest as default settings, and then select "START."

1. Press "d" on the keyboard to display the BO level.
2. Tell them to push the joystick in the direction where the small box is located (within the bigger box).
3. When the box goes double, ask the patient to blink and try to make the box back into one; if they cannot, they can wait for it to time out and bring it back down to a lower demand, or they can press random choices that will also bring it down to a lower level.
4. The BO goal is between 40 and 50 on this program.
5. Record the max goal achieved and also the recovery (once it doubled, determine at what level they brought it back to single).
6. Once they reached the max BO goal, let them work on base in (goal is 22 BI).
7. Once they have reached the BI goal, then let them work on jump ductions (the BO goal is 33, while the BI goal 18)

For convergence excess: Similar instructions are being followed as the aforementioned, but they may want to start with the "large size" to start and select "BI."

1. The BI goal is 25, while the BO goal is 40–50; then the jump ductions are BO goal 33 and BI goal 18.
2. Convergence excess (esophoria) patients tend to have trouble with RDS, so if they have trouble with this, go to the girl on the beach, or the frog, and choose a bigger target to start out with.
3. If the patient cannot do this; then go to "Vergence" and choose a flat fusion target (e.g., light bulbs). The patient can manually increase the BI demand by moving the joystick to the right.

RED/GREEN BARREL CARD (FIGURE 8.4)

Purpose

To improve convergence recovery ability

Equipment

- Barrel card

Set-up

- Instruct the patient to hold the red/green barrel card with their thumb and index finger at the bottom edge, midway between the front and back edge.
- Direct the patient to place the card directly straight in front of their nose with the smallest barrel toward them and the largest barrel furthest from them.
- For them to check that the card is in the proper position and is not tilted, make them alternately wink each eye. If they see the same amount of card on each side, the card is properly placed.

Procedure

1. Instruct the patient to focus their eyes on the barrel furthest from their eye (the largest barrel) until they see it clearly and singly. While they look at the furthest barrel, the middle and closest barrel should be seen double.
2. Then have the patient look out to a distance target. The distance target should be seen as one image and they should now be aware of the two barrel cards that will appear to be parallel. Tell the patient to hold this focus for a count of 5.
3. Then direct the patient to shift their fixation to the middle barrel until they see it singly and clearly. Repeat the previous steps.
4. Finally, make the patient focus their eyes on the near barrel until it is single, while the other two are double.
5. Repeat these steps. Perform 10 jumps and 3 repetitions with a 1 minute rest between repetitions.

Notes

- Instruct the patient to shift their focus back and forth from the distance target to each barrel.
- Always make them sure that whatever barrel they fixate is clear and single and that the remaining ones are double.

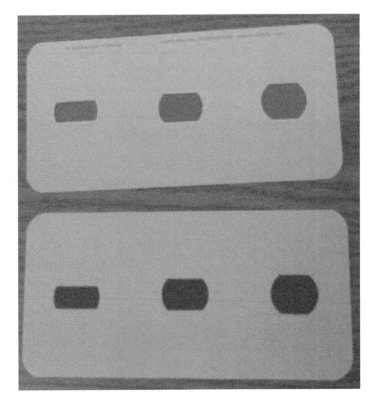

Figure 8.4 **(See color insert.)** Barrel card. (Courtesy of Bernell.com.)

- Tell the patient that if they *cannot* get the furthest barrel to become single, move the card away from their nose until they can and then start there.

Variations

- When instructed by the doctor, make the patient perform the procedure while balanced on a pillow.

POLARIZED FUSION SHEET (FIGURE 8.5)

Purpose

To work on convergence

Equipment

- Polaroid glasses
- Polaroid fusion sheet (on the next page)
  - Instruct the patient to put a pair of Polaroid glasses on themselves.
  - Direct the patient to close their left eye and take a piece of a Polaroid glass and position

it (turn it) in a way that they can see the top arrow underneath it and then tape it on to the page. To double-check, let them flip it the other way; it should now look black.
- Have the patient close their right eye and take a piece of Polaroid glass and position it so they can see the bottom arrow underneath it. Then let them tape it on to the page.
- Now with both eyes opened, they should see both arrows; if not, they need to go through the steps again. Their right eye should see the top arrow only, while their left eye should see the bottom arrow only.
- Prism
- Rx glasses

Duration

10 minutes

Set-up

- Instruct the patient to hold the Polaroid fusion sheet 16″ away from the front of the patient.
- Direct the patient to put on the Polaroid glasses.

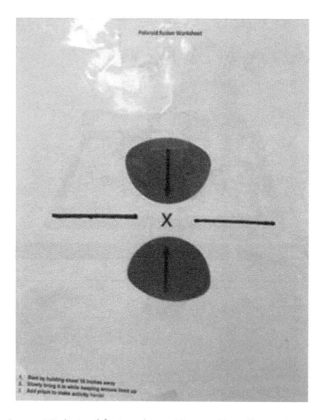

Figure 8.5 **(See color insert.)** Polarized fusion sheet. (Created by Allen Cohen.)

- To address convergence, make the patient move the Polaroid sheet slowly toward their face while keeping the arrows lined up.
- To address divergence, let the patient move the Polaroid sheet away from their face while keeping the arrows lined up.

Variations

Add a BI or BO prism to increase the difficulty.

- Place a prism in front of the eye. Line arrows back up.
- Take the prism away and add it back, keeping the arrows line up.

POLARIZED FUSION SHEET

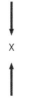

Clown vectogram (Figure 8.6)

Purpose

To improve vergence ranges and third-degree fusion

Equipment

- Clown vectogram and vectogram holder
- Polarized glasses
- Pointer

Set-up

- Instruct the patient to place the clown vectogram in the holder at the patient's eye level and then set it to @ (zero).
- Have the patient seated approx. 18″, away from the vectogram.
- Have the patient put on the glasses.
- Note that the numbers are for the BO ranges, while the letters are for BI ranges.

Procedure

1. Instruct the patient to look at the clown and to see the whole picture as clear and single.

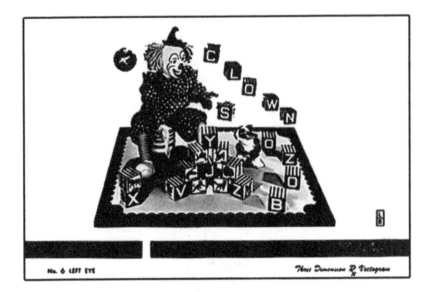

Figure 8.6 Clown vectogram. (Courtesy of Bernell.com.)

2. Have the patient get started by separating the vectogram slowly to either numbers or letters depending on the patient's binocular disorder.
3. Ask the patient to let you know when it becomes blurry or double.
   a. If it becomes blurry, tell them to try to clear it before you continue; if they cannot perform this, go back 2 units and continue to step 4.
   b. If it becomes double, tell them to try to make it single; if they cannot do this, go back 2 units and continue to step 4
4. Ask them if they can see the clown clear and single. If they still cannot do this, go back to where they can and record that number; this is their recovery.
5. Ask them if they noticed that some of the blocks are floating closer to them than others and if it looks 3D (this is floating).
6. Ask them to take the pointer and point to a block, where it is in space (this is localization).
   a. If they are able to do this, they will see one pointer and one letter.
   b. If they see two pointers and one letter, have them move the pointer slightly back and forth until they have one pointer and one letter.

   c. If they see two letters and one pointer, tell them to take the pointer away and get the letter back into one and then try again.
   d. Tell them that the closer they are to the letter, the closer the two pointers will be to each other and that the further away they are to the letter, the further away they will be.
7. Once they are able to localize, you want them to keep the pointer on the letter and to separate the vectogram again and ask them to keep one letter and one pointer.
8. The goal is to maximize out BI and BO.

Notes

- When they have reached approx. halfway to their goal, have them look away from the vectogram and look back and get it back into one. This is called "lookaways."
- When they have reached approx. halfway to their goal, also measure the opposite range, i.e., if they have convergence insufficiency and you are training BO ranges, once they get to ~18, also train BI ranges.
- When they have reached their goal, you want them to keep the vectogram single while they turn their head (left, right, up, and down).

SPIRANGLE VECTOGRAM (FIGURE 8.7)

Purpose

To improve vergence ranges and third-degree fusion, making it more challenging than the clown vectogram since the letters are further separated in space, which is good for training BO

Equipment

- Spirangle vectogram and vectogram holder
- Polarized glasses
- Pointer

Set-up

- Instruct the patient to place the vectogram in the holder at the patient's eye level and set it to @ (zero).
- Have the patient seated approx. 18″ away from the vectogram.
- Have the patient put on the glasses.
- Note that the numbers are for BO ranges, while the letters are for BI ranges.

Procedure

1. Follow the same procedure as that with the clown vectogram but want them to jump between letters; the inner ones are further away (less BO demand) and the outer ones are closer to the patient (more BO demand).

CLOWN/SPIRANGLE VECTOGRAM JUMP DUCTIONS (FIGURE 7.7)

Set-up

- Instruct the patient to place the clown vectogram on the top vectogram holder; this will be for BI.
- Also, direct the patient to place the spirangle vectogram on the bottom vectogram holder; this will be for BO.

Procedure

1. Let the patient slide the clown to C and slide the spirangle to 3.
2. Have the patient start by looking at the clown, keep it clear and single, and then jump to the spirangle and keep in single. Do this back and forth three times.
3. Direct the patient to slide the clown to F and slide the spirangle to 6.
4. Repeat step 2, and so on, and so forth.
5. Ask them if they see a size difference between the clown and the spirangle: BI should look larger, while BO should look smaller.

ECCENTRIC CIRCLE CONVERGENCE (FIGURE 8.8)

Purpose

To help develop the coordination and focusing ability of the patient's eyes when they look at near objects

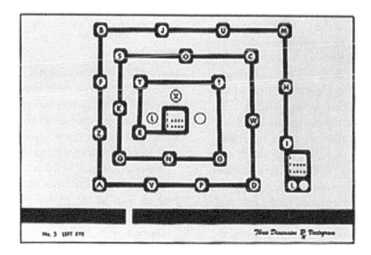

Figure 8.7 Spirangle vectogram. (Courtesy of Bernell.com.)

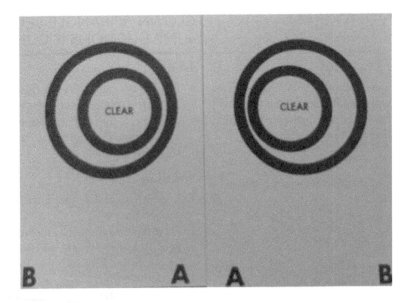

Figure 8.8 Eccentric circles. (Courtesy of Bernell.com.)

Equipment

- Eccentric circles
- Pencil

Procedure 1

1. Have the patient seated comfortably with good posture. Instruct them to hold the cards at 13″–16″ away from their eyes and then overlap A with A.
2. Direct the patient to hold a pencil, centered between the lower edges of the circles. Make them look directly at the tip of the lead and observe the circles on either side without looking directly at them.
3. Make them slowly move the pencil toward their nose (always looking at the tip and keeping it single) until they see four circles.
4. Let them continue the procedure by moving the pencil toward their nose. Let them observe the inner two circles approach each other until they see them overlap and superimposed. The patient should then see three circles: one to the right, one to the left, and one in the middle above their pencil tip. Direct them to stop moving their pencil at this point.
5. The middle circle should appear to have a 3D effect with the outer circle floating closer to them; it should also appear smaller and closer than the original two circles. This is fusion.

6. Next, tell the patient to try to clear the letters on the middle circle. When this can be done, let them try removing the pencil without moving their eyes and see if the middle circle can be maintained.

Procedure 2

Instruct the patient to repeat procedure 1 without the aid of a pencil. When the patient can easily fuse the circles without a pencil, have them begin tromboning the card near (toward their nose) and far (away at arm's length). At all times, keep the letters clear and in constant fusion.

Procedure 3

Direct the patient to look at a detailed distant target (calendar, clock, etc. more than 10′ away) and make it clear. Then make them look at the card, fuse the circles, and clear and notice the depth of the middle circle. Have them repeat this until they can easily look from a distant target to the cards with fusion.

No pencil is used in this exercise. Tell the patient to remember to clear the distant target and then look at near to the lifesaver card for fusion and clarity, then back to the distant target, etc.

Always use your appropriate glasses as prescribed by the doctor.

Procedure 4

Add head turns while keeping the middle circle fused.

ECCENTRIC CIRCLE DIVERGENCE

Purpose

To help develop the coordination and focusing ability of your eyes when you look at near objects and when you look from far to near objects

Equipment

- Clear eccentric circle cards
- Pencil

Procedure 1

1. Have the patient seated comfortably with good posture. Instruct them to hold the cards at 13″–16″ from their eyes and overlap A with A.
2. Make them center the pencil behind the card and then fixate and focus on the tip of the pencil as they move the pencil away from the card (i.e., further from them) until they see four circles. Have the patient try to feel their eyes turning out as they maintain focus.
3. Let them observe the inner two circles approach each other until they see the circles overlap and superimpose. The patient should then see three circles: one to the left, one to the right, and one in the middle, which should appear in 3D form with the inner circle floating closer to them. They should also appear larger and further away than the original two eccentric circles.
4. When this can be done, let them try removing the pencil without moving their eyes and see if the middle eccentric circle can be maintained.
5. Direct the patient to repeat the same procedure without using the pencil at all.

Procedure 2

1. Instruct the patient to repeat procedure 1, without the aid of a pencil. When they can easily fuse the circles without a pencil, let them begin tromboning the card near (toward their nose) and far (away at arm's length). At all times keep the letters clear and in constant fusion.

Procedure 3

1. Instruct the patient to look at a detailed distant target (calendar, clock, etc. more than 10′ away from them) and make it clear. Then make them look at the card, fuse the circles, and clear and notice the depth of the middle circle.

2. Have the patient repeat this until they can easily look from a distant target to the card with fusion and clarity, then back to the distant target, etc.

LIFESAVER CARD CONVERGENCE TECHNIQUE (FIGURE 8.9)

Purpose

To help develop the coordination and focusing ability of the eyes when they look at near objects and when they look from far to near objects

Equipment

- Lifesaver card
- Pencil

Procedure 1

1. Have the patient seated comfortably with good posture. Instruct them to hold the card at 13″–16″ away from their eyes. Tell them to use

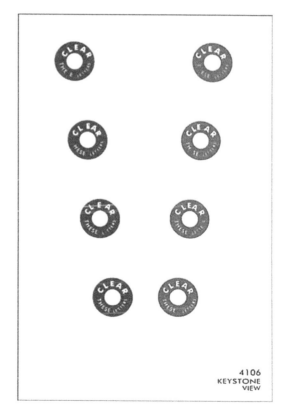

Figure 8.9 **(See color insert.)** Lifesaver card. (Courtesy of Bernell.com.)

only the bottom set of lifesavers on the card. It is helpful to cover the other sets with a sheet of white paper.

2. Make them hold a pencil, centered between the lower edges of the bottom circles and look directly at the tip of the lead; let them observe the circles on either side without looking directly at them.

3. Direct them to slowly move the pencil toward their nose (always looking at the tip and keeping it single) until they see four circles.

4. Have them continue moving the pencil toward their nose. Let them observe the inner two circles approach each other until they see them overlap and superimpose. The patient should then see three circles: one red, one green, and the one in the middle above their pencil tip. Make them stop moving their pencil at this point.

5. The middle circle should appear to be a different color than either the red or the green of the other lifesavers. It should also appear smaller and closer than the original two lifesavers. This is fusion.

6. Next, let the patient try to clear the letters on the middle lifesaver. When this can be done, have them try removing the pencil without moving their eyes and see if the middle lifesaver can be maintained.

Procedure 2

Instruct the patient to repeat the earlier procedure, one at a time with the other circles on the lifesaver card, one set at a time.

Procedure 3

Direct the patient to repeat procedure 2 without the aid of a pencil. When they can easily fuse the circles without a pencil, let them begin tromboning the card near (toward their nose) and far (away at arm's length). At all times, have them keep the letters clear and in constant fusion.

Procedure 4

- Instruct the patient to look at a detailed distant target (calendar, clock, etc. more than 10′ away) and make it clear. Then have them look at the card, fuse the circles, and clear and notice the depth of the middle circle.
- Direct the patient to repeat this until they can easily look from a distant target to the cards with fusion.

- No pencil is used in this exercise. Tell the patient to remember to clear the distant target and then look at near to the lifesaver card for fusion and clarity, then back to the distant target, etc.

Always use your appropriate glasses as prescribed by the doctor.

LIFESAVER CARD DIVERGENCE

Purpose

To help develop the coordination and focusing ability of the eyes when they look at near objects and when they look from far to near objects

Equipment

- Clear lifesaver card
- Pencil

Procedure 1

1. Have the patient seated comfortably with good posture. Instruct the patient to hold the card at 13″–16″ away from their eyes. Have them use only the bottom set of lifesavers on the card. It is helpful to use paper clip in a blank white paper over the others.

2. Direct the patient to center the pencil behind the card and fixate and focus on the tip of the pencil as they move the pencil away from the card (i.e., further from them) until they see four circles. The patient should try to feel their eyes turning out as they maintain focus.

3. Let the patient observe the inner two circles approach each other until they see the circles overlap and superimpose. The patient should then see three circles: one red, one green, and one in the middle. The one in the middle should appear to be a different color than either the red or the green.

4. It should be a mixture of both colors and should also appear larger and further away than the two original lifesavers.

5. Next, let them try to clear the letters on the middle lifesaver. When this can be done, make them try removing the pencil without moving their eyes and see if the middle lifesaver can be maintained.

6. Have them repeat the same procedure without using the pencil at all.

Procedure 2

1. Instruct the patient to repeat the aforementioned procedure, one at a time with the other circles on the lifesaver card, one set at a time.

Procedure 3

1. Direct the patient to repeat procedure 2, without the aid of a pencil. When they can easily fuse the circles without a pencil, let them begin tromboning the card near (toward their nose) and far (away at arm's length). At all times, have them keep the letters clear and in constant fusion.

Procedure 4

1. Instruct the patient to look at a detailed distant target (calendar, clock, etc. more than 10′ away from them) and make it clear. Then make them look at the card, fuse the circles, and clear and notice the depth of the middle circle.
2. Have them repeat this until they can easily look from a distant target to the card with fusion and clarity, then back to the distant target, etc.

APERTURE RULE CONVERGENCE (FIGURE 8.10)

Purpose

To help improve the accuracy and efficiency of their two eyes working as a team and to coordinate this with the focusing ability of each eye

Equipment

- Aperture rule
- Red pointer stick

Set-up

- Instruct the patient to assemble the aperture rule with the AP card booklet placed at "0" on the scale and turn to the picture of the two clocks.
- Direct the patient to move the slider so that it is positioned at "1 and 2" on the scale.
- The patient should place the tip of their nose against the edge of the rule so they are looking through the slider window at the card.

Procedure

1. The patient should be instructed to close their right eye and the clock on the left will disappear; if they see part of a second clock, they should move the aperture rule slightly over to their right.
2. Next, the patient should close their left eye and the clock on the right will disappear. If they see part of a second clock, they should move the aperture rule slightly over to the left.
3. Now the patient should look at the picture with both eyes open and see one clock with one set of circles underneath it, with a cross above the circles and a dot below them. The picture should be clear and single. Remember that they

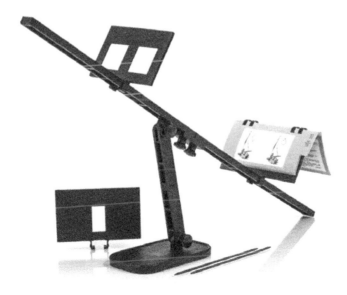

Figure 8.10 Aperture rule. (Courtesy of Bernell.com.)

must see both the cross and the dot at the same time. The circles should appear in 3D form.

4. If the patient cannot keep the targets single, place the red pointer stick next to the window opening. This will better orient the patient as to where their eyes should be looking.

5. When the patient is able to see one picture, they should look out into the distance and then back through the window slider; this should be performed several times, obtaining a clear single picture within a few seconds each time.

6. Now let the patient flip the card over to the two parrots (depending on which set you have) (AP 2). Have them keep the slider positioned where it is (1 and 2) and repeat steps 1 through 5. When they go to the next flip card (Golfer, AP 3), they will have to move the slider to position "3" on the scale. Just remember to always have the AP cards positioned at "0" but move the slider to the number on the scale that matches the AP card (slider to 4 on scale, for AP 4, and so on).

7. The goal is to get to card AP 12.

Guidelines

- There is no need to start with AP 1 each session; the patient can start with the card 3 steps back from where the patient last left off.
- The patient should not be discouraged if this is a tough procedure; it may take a while before they can attain the goal.

Note

- Once they are able to get to card AP 12, have them add a +1.00 lens flipper and have them do the same activity, and if they can do that, increase the power up to +2.00. (This modification is only for pre-presbyopic patients.)

APERTURE RULE DIVERGENCE

Purpose

To help improve the accuracy and efficiency of their two eyes working as a team and to coordinate this with the focusing ability of each eye

Equipment

- Aperture rule
- Red pointer stick

Set-up

- Instruct the patient to assemble the aperture rule with the AP card booklet placed at "0" on the scale and then turn to the picture of the two clocks.
- Make the patient move the slider so that it is positioned at "1 and 2" on the scale.
- Have the patient place the tip of their nose against the edge of the rule so that they are looking through the slider window at the card.

Procedure

1. The patient should be instructed to close their right eye and the clock on the left will disappear; if they see part of a second clock, they should move the aperture rule slightly over to their right.

2. Next, the patient should close their left eye and the clock on the right will disappear. If they see part of a second clock, they should move the aperture rule slightly over to the left.

3. Now, the patient should look at the target with both eyes open and should see one clock with one set of circles underneath it. The targets should be clear and single. Remember that they must see both the cross and the dot at the same time. The circles should appear in 3D form.

4. If they can't get or keep the targets single, let them place the red pointer in the hole of the rule, marked "A" on the scale. This will better orient the patient as to where their eyes should be looking; instruct the patient to take a deep breath and relax and look at the red pointer as if it were very far away.

5. Once they are able to see one picture, they should look over the flip card into the distance and then back through the window slider; they should be able to do this several times, obtaining a clear single picture within a few seconds each time they look back to the card.

6. Now instruct the patient to flip the card over to the two parrots (depending on which set they have) (AP 2). Have them keep the slider positioned where it its (1 and 2) and repeat steps 1 through 5. When they go to the next flip card (Golfer, AP 3), they will have to move the slider to position "3" on the scale. Just let them remember that always have the AP cards positioned at "0" but move the slider to the

number on the scale that matches the AP card (slider to 4 on scale, for AP 4, and so on).
7. The goal is to get to card AP 7.

Guidelines

- They should not be discouraged as this is a tough procedure, it may take a while before they can attain the goal. Even if they get to card AP 7, the speed with which they are able to see each picture as single and clear and the flexibility of being able to look away and look back again are more important.
- Remember that focusing outward and taking deep breaths will help with this exercise.

Note

- Once they are able to get to card AP 7, you may want to add a −1.00 lens flipper and have them do the same activity, and if they can do that, increase the power up to −2.00. (This modification is for pre-presbyopic patients)

POINTER IN THE STRAW

Purpose

To teach the two eyes to aim at a target and converge accurately

Equipment

Pointer or straighten paper clip
Straw

Duration

5–7 minutes

Set-up

- If you help with this procedure, you should hold the straw sideways (horizontal).
- However, if you do not assist in the procedure, then have the patient tape the straw sideways onto the side of a door.
- The straw should be at the eye level, 8″ away from the patient's nose.
- The patient should hold the pointer.

Instructions

1. Instruct the patient to look with both eyes at the straw opening and make sure they see it as single.
2. While keeping their eyes only on the straw, have them hold the pointer sideways and slowly move it closer to the straw.

3. The patient should be seeing the pointer only with their peripheral vision.
4. Once the patient is about 1″ away from the straw, direct them to take a pause, make one final adjustment, and put it in.
5. If they are able to do so, great; if not, let them start all the way back again.
6. The patient should do this 10 times.
7. Once this becomes easier for the patient, they can bring the straw closer to them by 1″ and start over again.

Notes

- The patient will be accurate only if their both eyes are open and working together; if it is too difficult, let them start with the straw further away.
- The patient can also move the straw above or below the eye level to challenge themselves.

DISTANCE ECCENTRIC CIRCLES (FIGURE 8.11)

Purpose

To teach the two eyes to converge voluntarily and be able to stabilize it while moving closer and further away from the target

Equipment

Large eccentric circles

Duration

5–7 minutes

Set-up

- Instruct the patient to make sure that they place the two sheets in line with each other and that one is not higher than the other.
- Direct the patient to make sure that the side with the smaller gap between the circles is pointing inward.
- Let them start by standing 6′ away from the center.

Instructions

1. Let the patient start the procedure by holding their finger approximately 8″ away, in line with their nose.
2. Have the patient look at the finger, and with their peripheral vision try to see a virtual third (middle) circle in between the two circles.

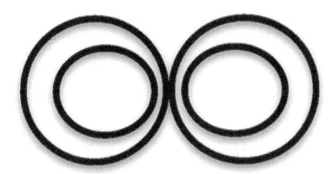

Figure 8.11 Distance eccentric circles.

3. Tell them to make sure the words CLEAR are clear and that the outer ring is floating toward them and the inner ring is receded.
4. If they do not see the third circle, let them try moving their finger slightly closer or further away until they are able to get it.
5. Once they are able to see the third circle, have them want to keep their eyes crossed at their finger, but slowly look at the circle. The goal is to take the finger away while still keeping the third circle.
6. Once the patient is able to do this, have them slowly walk closer and then further away, trying to keep the third circle the whole time.
7. The goal is to be as close as 4″ and as far as 12′ away.

Notes

- Add head rotations to make this more challenging.
- To make this a divergence activity, use clear acetate sheets and have someone walk behind the acetate sheets in order to get the third circle to appear.

VAN ORDEN STAR CONVERGENCE AND DIVERGENCE (FIGURE 8.12)

Purpose

To improve distance binocular stability with a motor task and to also work on antisuppression

Equipment

- Bernell Vision Trainer (bernell.com)
- Van Orden Star Sheets (oepf.org or bernell.com)
- Two sharpened pencils

Duration

5 minutes

Set-up

- The patient should be seated, looking into the viewfinder.
- The patient should hold a pencil in each hand.
- Esophoria patients should use the BI sheet, and exophoria patients should use the BO sheet

Directions

1. Instruct the patient to look into the viewfinder and be aware of the numbers on the left and right side of the sheet as well as the concentric circle in the center. They should be able to see depth in the circles.
2. The patient should then place the pencil on their left hand on the first number of the top left-hand corner.
3. Then they should place the pencil on their right hand on the last number of the bottom right-hand corner.
4. They should be instructed to keep their eyes on the center, but move the pencils toward each other (diagonally) until they look like they are touching, and then stop.
5. They should proceed to the next number (the second number from the top on the left side, the second number from the bottom on the right side), until they finish the sheet.
6. If one of the pencil tips disappears, they should stop and blink and then continue when the pencil tip reappears. If the center circle doubles

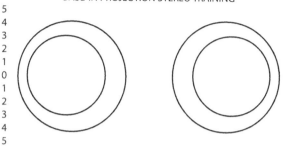

STAR THERAPY
FOR IMPROVEMENT OF BINOCULARITY AND FINE MOTOR SKILLS
BASE-IN PROJECTION STEREO TRAINING

Figure 8.12 Star therapy. (Courtesy of Bernell.com.)

or becomes "flat," they need to stop and blink and then continue when they are able to see one set of circles with depth.

Notes

- To see how accurate the patient was, the therapist should fold the sheet first so the vertical numbers on right and left side match up and then fold it again so the folded edge and the numbers match up.
- If the patient was able to perform accurately, the pencil lines that they drew should end on the second folded line from the center. If the pencil line does not reach the folded line, this is an underconvergence; if the pencil line crosses the folded line, this is an overconvergence.

Variations

- Add a BI or BO prism to make this task harder.

VERTICAL PRISM ALIGNMENT

Purpose

To train the eyes line up and stabilize when looking at a far distance

Equipment

- 1/4 sheet of the Hart chart or a 5″ × 5″ sheet of paper with some letters
- Prism of between 10 and 14 diopters

Set-up

- Place the small Hart chart on the wall at the patient's eye level.

- Have the patient stand approximately 8′ away from wall.
- Have the patient hold the prism base down in front of their right eye.

Instructions

1. Ask the patient if they see two charts on the wall and if they are lined up one directly above the other.
2. If they are lined up, excellent, have them take a step back and take a look again.
3. If they are not, ask the patient, "where is the top chart in respect to the bottom chart?"
   a. If the top chart is to the right, this is an esophoria drift
   b. If the top chart is to the left, this is an exophoria drift.
4. If it is an esophoria drift, ask the patient to try to relax their eyes, try to be more aware of their peripheral vision, and take a deep breath; also see if they can *make their eyes adjust* so that the top and the bottom line up.
5. If it is an exophoria drift, ask the patient to try to *concentrate* and *focus* their eyes, even *cross their eyes*, and see if they can make their eyes adjust so that the top and bottom line up.
6. If they can do so, follow step 2 and continue.
7. If they try the previous steps and they still cannot do it, try varying the distance between the patient and the chart, to see if there is a distance where it is easiest, and work from there.
8. If step 7 does not work, have the patient turn the prism slightly (clockwise if it is an exophoria drift and counterclockwise if it is an

esophoria drift) to see if it lines up. If this works, have them try to turn it back and still keep it lined up.

Notes

- This exercise is not suitable for all patients. This exercise is contraindicated for patients who have anomalous retinal correspondence.
- To make this exercise more challenging, you can have the patient rotate the prism slightly counterclockwise; this will misalign the chart and the patient will have to make the adjustment with their eyes to line up the chart again (for exophoria patients). Esophoria patients will rotate the prism clockwise.

MIRROR TRANSFER (FIGURE 8.13)

Purpose

To train the eyes to make accurate eye movement inward (convergence) and outward (divergence)

Equipment

- Two sheets of paper, one with a circle (o) and the other with a plus sign (+)
- A handheld mirror, preferably rectangular or square shaped

Set-up

- Find a corner of the room that is uncluttered.
- Have the patient stand facing one side of the wall (2′ away), with shoulder facing the other side of the wall (2′ away).
- Place the sheet with the "o" on the wall directly in front of the patient.
- Place the sheet with the "+" on the wall facing the patient's shoulder; they should be leveled.

Instructions

1. The patient should hold the mirror with both hands; the edge of the mirror should be resting on the bridge of their nose, and angle the mirror so that the patient can see the "+" in the "o."
2. Once the patient can see the overlapping images, have the patient slowly angle the mirror toward the wall until the "+" is slightly outside of the "o."
3. Now have the patient try to *relax* and *look through the wall in front of them*, so that the "+" goes back in the "o" (divergence).
4. Have the patient continue steps 2 through 3 until they can no longer overlap the two images
5. Once they are done with the earlier steps, have them "reset" by closing their eyes, then

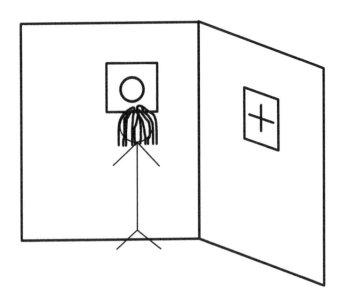

Figure 8.13 Mirror transfer set-up.

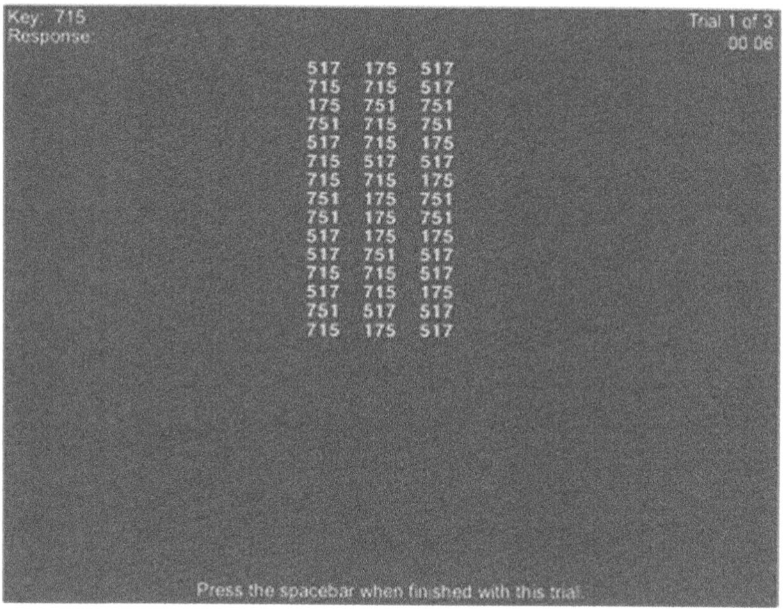

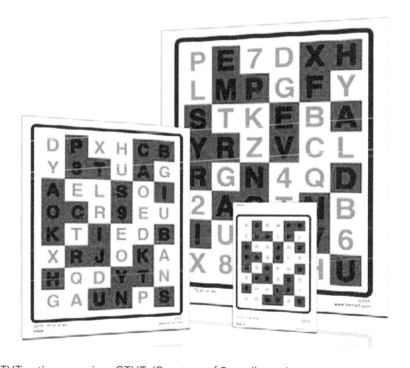

Figure 6.12 Computerized visual search. (Courtesy of Rodney K. Bortel.)

Figure 7.6 GTVT antisuppression: GTVT. (Courtesy of Bernell.com.)

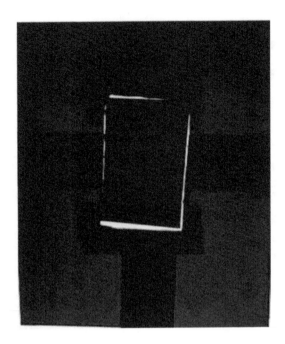

Figure 8.2 Cohen chart. (Created by Allen Cohen.)

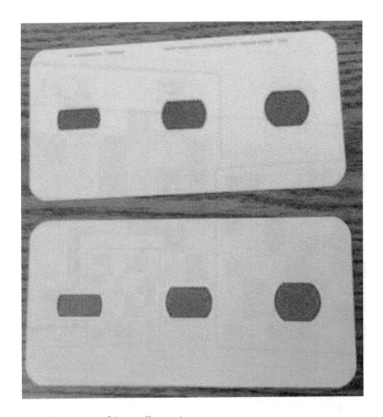

Figure 8.4 Barrel card. (Courtesy of Bernell.com.)

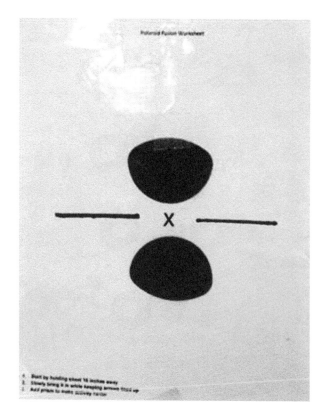

Figure 8.5 Polarized fusion sheet. (Created by Allen Cohen.)

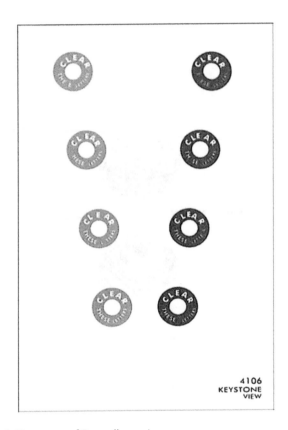

Figure 8.9 Lifesaver card. (Courtesy of Bernell.com.)

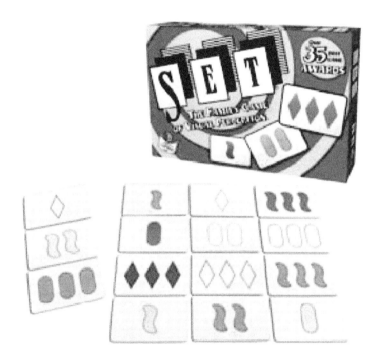

Figure 9.4 SET Dice®. (Courtesy of Cannei, LLC; Copyright © 1991.)

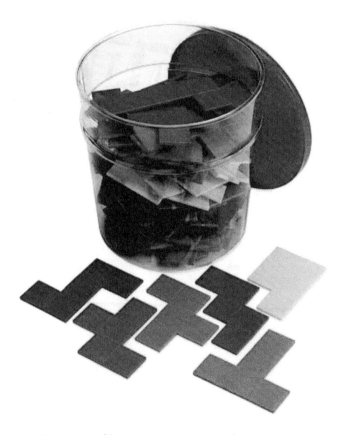

Figure 9.14 Pentaminoes. (Courtesy of learningresources.com.)

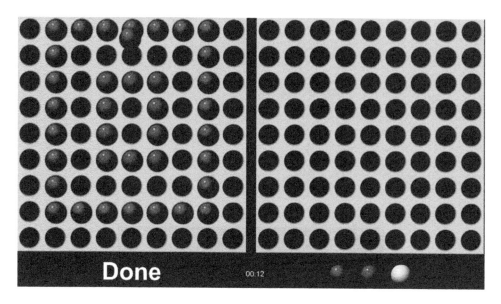

Figure 9.19 Computerized pegboard activity screen. (Courtesy of Rodney K. Bortel.)

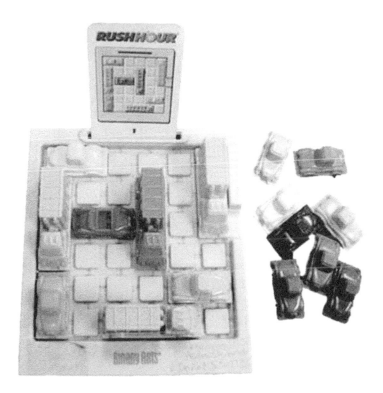

Figure 9.33 Rush Hour. (Courtesy of Thinkfun, Alexandria, VA.)

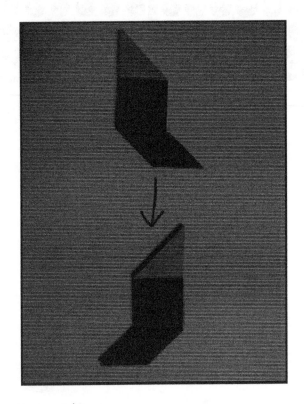

Figure 9.38 Parquetry pattern matching.

open them, and tilt the mirror to where the "+" and the "o" easily overlap.

6. Now have the patient slowly angle the mirror away from the wall until the "+" is slightly outside of the "o."

7. Have the patient try to *concentrate* and *cross* their eyes and have them *move their eyes* so that the "+" goes back in the "o" (convergence).

8. Have the patient continue steps 6 through 7 until they can no longer overlap the two images.

Notes

- It is important to note that convergence ability is naturally going to be much better than divergence ability.

- It is difficult to measure *norms* in this exercise because the angle changes that the patient makes are very small. In general, the patient wants to work on the area that gives them difficulty and overall improves their "range."

COLOR FUSION CARDS (FIGURE 8.14)

Purpose

To teach the two eyes to aim at a target accurately at distance and to work on antisuppression

Equipment

- Color fusion cards
- Stereoscope
- Two pointers

Duration

5–7 minutes

Set-up

- Slide the black holder to 0.00.
- Place the card centered on the holder.
- The patient should be wearing their distance glasses.
- The patient should have a pointer in each hand.

Instructions

1. Instruct the patient to look in the instrument at the card; they should see a center circle with arrows and it should be pointing at a red object.

2. If either the arrows or the red object disappears, have them blink and try to keep it from disappearing; sometimes tapping on it with a pointer helps.

3. Now direct them to look around at the letters, call them out, and, using both pointers, point them, making sure they are all single.

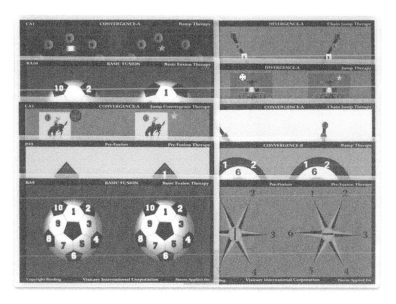

Figure 8.14 Color fusion cards. (Courtesy of Bernell.com.)

4. Have them move to card 2: now some of the letters should look in 3D form, making sure they are able to see them all singly again and point to each one with both pointers.

5. Each card after 2 has a slight variation, but all will be training the patient's ability to fuse the image from the right and left eye. Have the patient point to each target and have them maintain single vision.

9

Visual perception

Visual perception is the process of interpreting and integrating visual information with the other parts of the brain. From a neuroanatomical perspective, it is the connections that are made from the visual cortex to the visual association cortex. This includes the two commonly defined streams: One is the dorsal stream aka ambient system, "where" pathway that is responsible for producing our sense of spatial orientation, binocular fusion/depth perception, and the location, movement, movement direction and velocity of objects in space. The other is the ventral stream aka focal system, "what" pathway that is responsible for recognizing objects and colors, reading text, and learning and remembering visual objects.

Visual Perception in Mild Traumatic Brain Injury

Visual perceptual deficits can occur after mild traumatic brain injury (mTBI) but may be more subtle. mTBI slows the acquisition and processing of visual information, so naturally certain areas of visual perception, especially timed tests (i.e., visual processing speed), can be affected. Visual attention is another area that is affected in mTBI; therefore, visual discrimination and figure–ground can also be affected.

Visual Perception in Moderate-to-Severe TBI

Visual perceptual deficits in moderate-to-severe TBI are usually more focal and more severe. Injury to the parietal lobe will cause more deficits in the *where* pathway and will affect visual-motor integration. Injury to the temporal lobe will cause more deficits in the *what* pathway and will affect visual closure and visual discrimination.

The rest of this chapter will be defining the different visual perceptual processing areas and the different tests to identify them.

DESCRIPTION OF THE VISUAL PERCEPTUAL PROCESSING AREAS

There is more than one way to think of the hierarchy of visual processing skills. There is a certain amount of overlap and redundancy. What follows is one way to think of the relationship of these skills. As an example, some people consider visual spatial relations as its own entity, while others group it with visual analysis skills. For the most part, visual perceptual processing may be considered to have three component areas:

Visual Spatial Skills

- **Laterality**
  - This skill is an internal self-awareness of two body sides, knowing they are different and appropriately naming them as left or right.
- **Directionality**
  - This skill represents the ability to project left–right concepts into visual space, that is, the ability to evaluate left–right in a projected sense.
- **Bilateral integration**
  - The ability to use the two sides of the body either in unison or separately.

Visual Analysis Skills

- **Figure–ground**
  - This skill represents the ability to extract a particular piece of information while simultaneously ignoring or disregarding irrelevant information.

- **Visual discrimination**
  - This is the ability to identify the differences in features and forms such as shape, size, orientation, color, or any other quality.
- **Form constancy**
  - This skill allows the individual to consistently recognize an object despite changes in some of its properties such as size and orientation. This ability may be considered a subset of visual discrimination.
- **Visual spatial relations**
  - This skill represents the ability to understand directional concepts that organize visual space. These skills allow an individual to develop spatial concepts, such as right and left, front and back, and up and down, as they relate to their body and to objects in space.
- **Visual closure**
  - Visual closure is the ability to identify an incomplete object. This skill allows an individual to use a limited amount of visual information to determine the identity of a partial hidden or obscured object.
- **Visual spatial memory**
  - Visual spatial memory involves recalling the spatial location of a previously presented visual stimulus.
- **Visual sequential memory**
  - The ability to recall a sequence (objects, letters, numbers, or words etc.) in the order in which they were first displayed.
- **Processing speed**
  - This represents how quickly information is absorbed and utilized. It refers to both the speed of acquisition and the rate at which a simple visual task may be performed.
- **Visualization**
  - A higher-level skill needed to create a mental image of an object one has seen and then manipulate the image in his mind. In many ways, this skill is the culmination of all of the previously described visual abilities.

Visual Integration Skills:

- This skill represents the ability to coordinate visual input and processing with motor output. This includes both fine and gross motor (Figure 9.1).

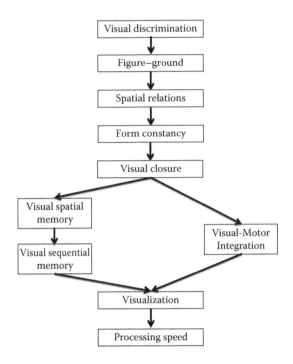

VISUAL PERCEPTUAL TESTING BATTERY

Before deciding on a course of treatment, a full visual perceptual assessment should be performed. In most ways, a visual perceptual assessment on a TBI patient is no different than the one performed on a learning disabled patient of the same age. A test or test battery should have the following characteristics:

- It should be reliable:
  - The test should give the same result if repeated on the same person.
  - The test should give the same result if repeated on the same person by a different examiner.
- It should demonstrate validity:
  - The test should measure what it purports to measure.

A comprehensive battery should include testing for all major areas of visual perceptual processing. Generally, this is accepted to encompass visual spatial orientation skills, visual analysis skills, and visual integration skills. Not all test batteries contain all of the elements that one would like to have tested for a TBI patient. For this population, a full battery should include

	Visual discrimination	Visual figure–ground	Visual spatial relations	Visual form constancy	Visual closure	Visual-motor integration	Visual spatial memory	Visual sequential memory	Visualization	Perceptual speed
Differences/Differix	1°	2°	2°							
Visual Discrimination workbook	1°	2°	2°						2°	
Jigsaw Puzzles	1°	1°	1°	1°	1°				1°	
SET		1°		1°					1°	
Spot-It		1°		2°						
I SPY Eagle Eye		1°		2°						
Visual Perceptual Speed (CPT)	2°	1°	2°							1°
Visual Scan (CPT)	2°	1°								
Visual Search (CPT)	2°	1°	2°							1°
Word Search		1°			2°					
Hidden Pictures		1°		2°						
Katamino			1°							
Tangrams/Tangoes			1°							
Geoboard/Rosner Patterns			1°	2°						
Rubber Road GEO shapes			1°	2°						
Pentominoes/Parquetry			1°	2°						
Pegboard activities			1°	2°						
Pegboard (CPT)			1°							
Duplo			1°	2°						
Soma cubes			1°	2°						
Colorku			1°	2°						
Visual Closure (CPT)	2°				1°					
Dot to Dot	2°				1°	1°				

(Continued)

Figure 9.1 A proposal for the sequencing of visual perceptual therapy for the TBI patient.

	Visual discrimination	Visual figure–ground	Visual spatial relations	Visual form constancy	Visual closure	Visual-motor integration	Visual spatial memory	Visual sequential memory	Visualization on	Perceptual speed
Creating Line Design Books	2°			2°		1°				
Developing Visual-Motor Integration	2°					1°				
Visual Concentration (CPT)			2°				1°		2°	
Improving Visual Memory Unit 1/1°			2°				1°		1°	
Tic-tac-toe with memory component			2°				1°			
Parquetry Pattern Matching			1°				1°		1°	
Visual Sequential Processing (CPT)								1°		
Visual Span (CPT)								1°		
Visual Memory (CPT)							1°	1°		2°
Rush Hour				2°				1°	1°	
SUNY Visual-Motor Forms							1°			1°
Visual Coding (CPT)										1°
Tachistoscope (CPT)										1°

Figure 9.1 (Continued) A proposal for the sequencing of visual perceptual therapy for the TBI patient.

- Visual discrimination
- Visual spatial relations
- Visual closure
- Visual form constancy
- Visual figure–ground
- Visual-motor integration
- Fine motor
- Visual sequential memory
- Visual spatial memory

It is essential that the testing is performed by a qualified practitioner. Many tests of good reliability and validity are available. Care should be taken to be sure that the age range for a given test is appropriate for the patient. Some commonly used tests are described here:

- **Developmental Test of Visual Perception, Adolescent and Adult (DTVP-A)**
  - The age range is 11.0–74.11 years.
  - This includes six subtests:
    - Copying
    - Figure–ground
    - Visual-motor search
    - Visual closure
    - Visual-motor speed
    - Form constancy
  - It takes approximately 25 minutes to administer.
  - The sections may be given and scored individually.
  - This gives a composite score (index) for three areas:
    - General visual perceptual index
    - Motor-reduced visual perception index
    - Visual-motor integration index
- **Developmental Test of Visual Perception, Third Edition (DTVP-3)**
  - The age range is 4.0–12.11 years.
  - This includes five subtests:
    - Copying
    - Figure–ground
    - Eye–hand coordination
    - Visual closure
    - Form constancy
  - It takes approximately 30 minutes to administer.
  - The sections may be given and scored individually.

- It gives a composite score (index) for three areas:
  - Motor-reduced visual perception
  - Visual-motor integration
  - General visual perception
- **Test of Visual Perceptual Skills, Third Edition (TVPS-3)**
  - The age range is 4.0–18.11 years.
  - This includes seven subtests:
    - Visual discrimination
    - Visual memory
    - Visual spatial relationships
    - Visual form constancy
    - Visual sequential memory
    - Visual closure
    - Visual figure–ground takes approximately 10–20 minutes to administer.
  - The sections may be given and scored individually.
  - This gives scaled scores and percentile ranks.
  - It does not have a motor component.
- **Beery-Buktenica Developmental Test of Visual-Motor Integration, 6th Edition (BEERY™ VMI)**
  - The age range is 2–100 years (ages 19 and up have not been updated since 2006).
  - This takes approximately 15 minutes to administer.
  - It gives standard scores and percentiles.
  - This is a good test to utilize when the TVPS-3 is used.
  - It has three components:
    - BEERY VMI
    - Motor coordination
    - Visual perception
- **PTS test, Computerized Perceptual Therapy Assessment**
  - The age range is 6.0–13.11 years.
  - This gives scaled scores and percentiles.
  - It has three components:
    - Tachistoscope (speed of information processing)
    - Visual span (visual sequential processing)
    - Visual closure (visual simultaneous processing)

DISCRIMINATION

Differences/Differix (Figures 9.2 and 9.3)

Purpose

- To develop visual attention and visual discrimination as a precursor for more sophisticated, that is, higher-level visual perceptual processes

Equipment

- Differences or Differix cards and pattern boards

Set-up

- The patient sits with good posture before the pattern board.
- Some cards are more complicated and with more details.
- Start with the most basic pattern (as required).

Procedure

1. The patient is told that each card can only be placed over one specific picture on the pattern board.
2. The patient must compare each card and place it over the appropriate pattern board picture.

3. If necessary, have the patient verbally describe the card to help reinforce the visual system with auditory support.
4. Each card has an overlay to show the correct answers.
5. If necessary, remove any incorrectly placed cards and have the patient retry for the correct placement.

Notes

- The clinician can help improve the patient's abilities by providing strategies.
- The patient can be taught to look for relevant information and exclude the irrelevant. This skill will be further developed in the figure–ground section.
- Document the pattern, number of retries, and speed if timed.
- This is ideally an office-based technique.

Variations

- Time the patient as the skill develops to improve automaticity.
- Have the patient start in the top left of the pattern card and work from left to right and top to bottom to further develop organizational skills.

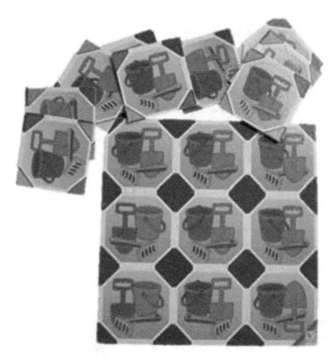

Figure 9.2 Differences game. (Courtesy of Ravensburg, Newton, NH.)

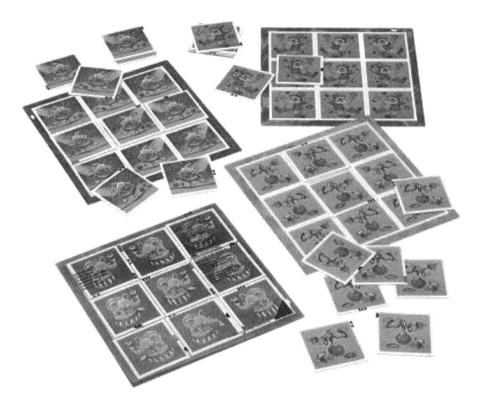

Figure 9.3 Proposal for the sequencing of visual perceptual therapy for the TBI patient. (Courtesy of Differix by Ravensburg, Newton, NH.)

Availability

- Amazon.com

Visual discrimination workbook

Purpose

- Office and home exercise to further the development of visual discrimination skills

Equipment

- Visual discrimination workbook

Procedure

1. The patient looks at the picture pair that sets "the rule." The rule is a picture pair that has performed a spatial transformation. Now the patient must apply this rule to find the correct picture in the trial that follows the same rule.
2. Patient should ideally complete one to two pages per day.
3. Patient should be told to emphasize accuracy over speed.
4. Patient can check for correctness as answers are printed at the back of the book.

Notes

- The procedure can be repeated with timing if desired.
- The patient could be advised to add an auditory support component by verbally describing the target image.

Variations

- The procedure can be repeated as a timed exercise if desired.

Availability

- Jean Edwards (author)
- Publisher: Didax
- Available from the following websites:
  - Amazon.com
  - www.therapro.com

Jigsaw puzzles

Purpose

- To develop shape and color discrimination skills while also promoting visualization, form perception, visual closure, and figure–ground

Equipment

- Simple puzzles should be used at first.
- Depending on the patient's needs and abilities, puzzles may need to be no more than 25 pieces at first.
- As skills develop, number of pieces can increase. As therapy proceeds and the more advance visual perception skills are attended to, puzzle size can go up to as much as 500 pierces.

Set-up

- Patient should devote an ample space that will not be disturbed throughout the duration of the home exercise.

Procedure

1. Based on the patient's level of abilities and stamina, he should be asked to place as few or as many pieces per night as the clinician feels is appropriate.
2. Work in a quiet room with appropriate lighting.

Notes

- Puzzles should be carefully selected.
- At first, the better choice of picture design would be large pieces with bold colors and high contrast between the patterns on each piece.

- Later, a more challenging picture would be subtle variations in shade with minimal contrast between patterns.
- Ideally a home technique but can be used in office.

Visual figure–ground (Figures 9.4 and 9.5)

Purpose

- To develop skills that help distinguish an object from the background in an array or, more exactly, to pull out relevant visual information from the irrelevant
- To be very useful in developing cognitive flexibility by rapidly switching task goals
- To be used in an office or at home

Equipment

- SET® cards

Set-up

- After carefully mixing the "deck" of SET cards, lay out 20 cards in 4 rows and 5 columns.
- The clinician must be sure he or she has dealt out at least one *SET*.

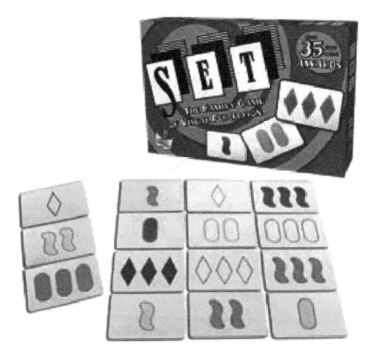

Figure 9.4 **(See color insert.)** SET Dice®. (Courtesy of Cannei, LLC; Copyright © 1991.)

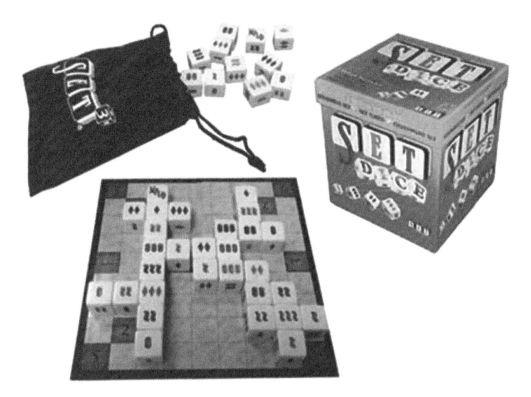

Figure 9.5 SET Dice®. (Courtesy of Cannei, LLC; Copyright © 1991.)

Procedure

1. Each card has pictures with four attributes:
   a. Color, number, shape, and filling.
2. The goal is to find a series of three cards where for each attribute the cards are all different or all the same.
3. Once a *SET* of three cards is found, they are removed from the array and replaced with three more.

Notes

- Dealing out more cards increases the likelihood of finding a *SET* but also increases the visual figure–ground confusion.

Variations

- SET Dice (latest variation)
- To make the task easier:
  - One color can be removed from the deck to limit the variables to 3 rather than 4.
  - The clinician can choose two cards and ask the patient to describe the card that is needed to complete the *SET* (there can only be only one card if two have already been chosen).
- Timing can be added for higher-level patients.

I SPY Eagle Eye™

Purpose

- To develop skills that help distinguish an object from the background in an array or, more exactly, to pull out relevant visual information from the irrelevant
- To be also very useful in developing cognitive flexibility by rapidly switching task goals
- To be used in an office or at home

Equipment

- I SPY Eagle Eye™ game

Set-up

- A given game board is placed before the patient along with a single game card.

Procedure

1. The patient is told that for a given game board there will be one and only one picture on the game card to be found on the board.
2. He should be helped to develop a strategy to find the correct item.

3. Some game boards have "themes," so the patient should be encouraged to look for the theme-related items first.

Notes

- Some board–card combinations are faster than others. The clinician must use his judgment when deciding if a patient is truly mastering this concept.
- Some game boards are easier than others due to less elements or larger elements. Take the patient's abilities into account when selecting the game board.

Variations

- Timing can be used for higher-level patients, though rarely done in practice.
- I SPY Eagle Eye Jr. Game (simpler version) for lower-level patients.
- Spot-it is an even more simplified variation of the technique.
- The technique can be made much easier by the clinician finding the answer and telling the patient the specific item on the card that they need to find.

Availability

- Amazon.com

Visual perceptual speed: CPT (Figures 9.6 and 9.7)

Purpose

- To develop skills that help distinguish an object from the background in an array or, more exactly, to pull out relevant visual information from the irrelevant
- To develop improved scanning skills and quickly recognize visual information
- To help further develop saccadic accuracy

Equipment

- CPT computer program

Set-up

- The patient is seated at the appropriate distance from the computer screen (based on screen size).
- Appropriate parameters are entered based on the patient's needs and abilities.

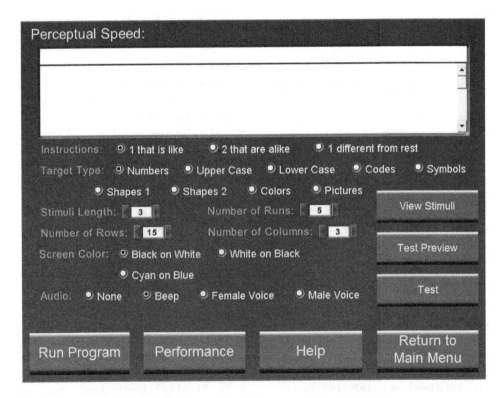

Figure 9.6 Visual perceptual speed set-up screen. (Courtesy of Bernell.com.)

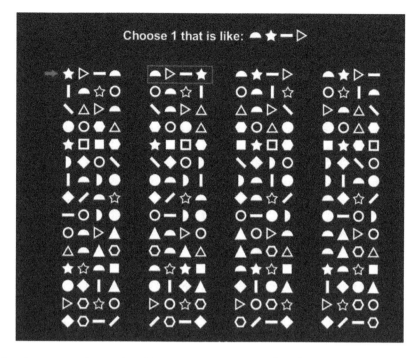

Figure 9.7 Visual perceptual speed activity screen. (Courtesy of Rodney K. Bortel.)

- The parameters include
  - Number of elements
  - Number of columns
  - Type of elements, i.e., numbers, letters, simple or complex shapes, pictures, and colors
  - Whether to search for the one alike, one different, or two alike targets

Procedure

1. *For "one different"*: The patient is told to find the one target different from the others.
2. *For "one alike"*: The patient is told to correctly match the template on top with the same sequence in the row marked by an arrow.
3. *For "two alike"*: Two patients are told to find the two sequences that are alike within the marked row. There is no top template.
4. These are ordered in increasing difficulty.

Notes

- Increased difficulty results from
  - Increased number of elements and columns
  - Progressing from numbers, letters, simple to complex shapes, pictures, and colors

  - More organized visual search CPT program as it can be used to promote left to right visual attack
- This technique was originally intended to be timed. This needs only to be done with more advanced patients; however, reasonable accuracy should always be stressed.

Availability

- http://www.visiontherapysolutions.net

Visual scan: CPT/PTS II (Figures 9.8 and 9.9)

Purpose

- To develop skills that help distinguish an object from the background in an array or, more exactly, to pull out relevant visual information from the irrelevant
- To develop improved scanning skills and quickly recognize visual information
- To help further develop saccadic accuracy

Equipment

- CPT computer program

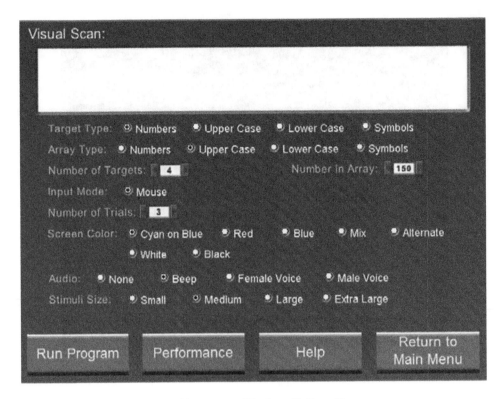

Figure 9.8 Visual scan set-up screen. (Courtesy of Rodney K. Bortel.)

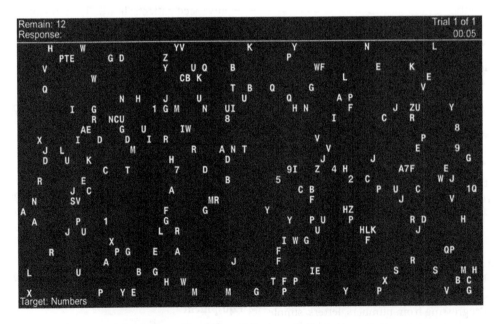

Figure 9.9 Visual scan activity screen. (Courtesy of Rodney K. Bortel.)

Set-up

- The patient is seated at the appropriate distance from the computer screen (based on screen size).
- Appropriate parameters are entered based on the patient's needs and abilities.
- The parameters include
  - *Target*: Number and type (numbers, upper- or lowercase letters, symbols)
  - *Array*: Number and type (numbers, upper- or lowercase letters, symbols)
  - *Size of screen elements*: Small, medium, or large
  - *Screen colors*: A variety available

Procedure

1. The goal is to find the targets embedded in an array of distractors.
2. The patient selects the target with the mouse.

Notes

- The greater the number or targets, the easier the task.
- The greater the number in the background array, the harder the task.

- This technique is timed but timing may be disregarded to stress accuracy.
- This is available for home use on the PTS II system.

Variations

- Based on the patient's other visual needs, this task may be performed monocularly or when properly set up with red/blue glasses for fusion needs.
- This is available for home use on PTS II program though with minimal parameter control. The computer will increase difficulty as the patient progresses.

Availability

- http://www.visiontherapysolutions.net

Visual search: CPT/PTS II (Figures 9.10 and 9.11)

Purpose

- To develop skills that help distinguish an object from the background in an array or,

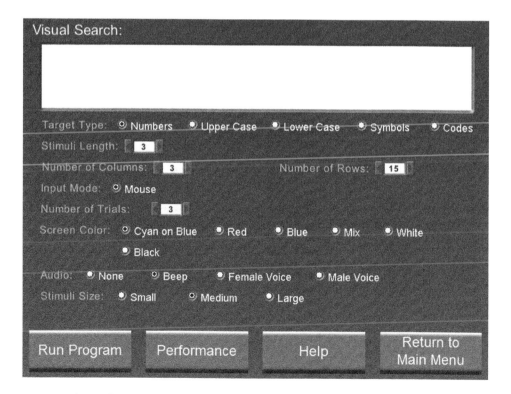

Figure 9.10 Visual search set-up screen. (Courtesy of Rodney K. Bortel.)

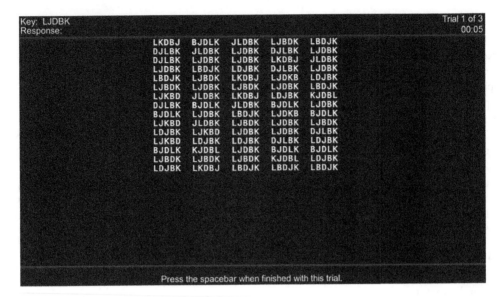

Figure 9.11 Visual search activity screen. (Courtesy of Rodney K. Bortel.)

- more exactly, to pull out the relevant visual information from the irrelevant
- To develop improved scanning skills and quickly recognize visual information

Equipment

- CPT computer program

Set-up

- Based on the patient's needs and abilities, the clinician sets the length and type of stimulus as well as the number of columns and rows.

Procedure

1. The patient is asked to locate all copies of the key (found in the upper-left part of the screen) in the array.
2. When the patient feels they have found them all, they press the space bar.

Notes

- The patient should be helped to develop strategies as needed to be sure to find all the targets. Auditory support is often helpful.

Variations

- This is available for home use on PTS II program though with minimal parameter control. The computer will increase difficulty as the patient progresses.

Availability

- http://www.visiontherapysolutions.net

Home figure–ground techniques

Jigsaw Puzzles

- As described in section "Visual Discrimination"

Word Search

- Clinician may assign this exercise by the selection of preprinted books.
- Many computer-based programs are available online (freeware).
- All the following are printable. Ideally, the clinician should make a supply of samples of different degrees of difficulty to hand out in advance:
  - http://www.toolsforeducators.com/wordsearch/
  - http://puzzlemaker.discoveryeducation.com/WordSearchSetupForm.asp
  - http://www.puzzle-club.com/free-printable-word-searches-themes1.html

Hidden Pictures

- Many books are available from Amazon.com, Inc., Barnes & Noble (bn.com), and others
- Online-based programs

- Note these go from easy to hard; the clinician must choose the appropriate level of difficulty:
  - http://www.games.com/hidden-object-games (online only)
  - http://www.highlightskids.com/hidden-pictures/interactive/archive#

Notes

- All home techniques must be attempted in the office first. There is no value in the patient going home just to discover they could not perform the exercise or did not understand the instructions.

Spatial relations (Figure 9.12)

Purpose

- To develop the ability to perceive the position of objects in relation to oneself and other objects
- To be used in an office or at home

Equipment

- Katamino (older version): 10, 5 unit shapes plus smaller pieces
- Katamino Deluxe: 12, 5 unit shapes
  - Both game designs have appropriate uses.

Set-up

- The clinician sets wooden game board before the patient.
- Choose basic or advanced set based on the patient's abilities (see "Notes").
- Explain the task to the patient.
- Start at the most basic level and add difficulty as needed.

Procedure

1. A wooden divider slide is placed in the appropriate slot; #3 is ideal for first-time use.
2. The patient is told to use the specific pieces to fill in the empty block of the puzzle.

Notes

- For lower-level patients, the 10 + 5 version can be ideal as the task can be simplified by using the 1 × 1 or 1 × 2 pieces.
- The technique tends to get very hard quickly.
- No one will be able to achieve all levels.

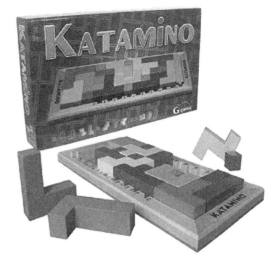

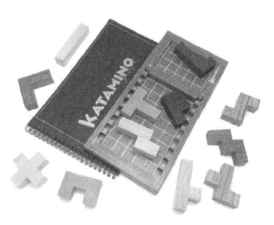

Figure 9.12 Katamino. (Courtesy of Gigamic.)

Variations

- If the task is becoming too difficult, for example, at level 5, the clinician can perform a technique called "level 5—any piece." This would ask the patient to complete the 5 × 5 grid using any pieces the patient chooses. If successful, the clinician removes one piece from the grid and now the patient must use any five of the remaining pieces.

Availability

- Amazon.com

Tangrams/Tangoes (Figure 9.13a)

Purpose

- To develop the ability to perceive the position of objects in relation to oneself and other objects
- To be used as a tool for improving visualization
- To be used in an office or at home

Equipment

- Any of the varied commercially available tangram sets
- Premade patterns, useful but not mandatory and very much available
- Small and large sizes, available based on the patient's needs

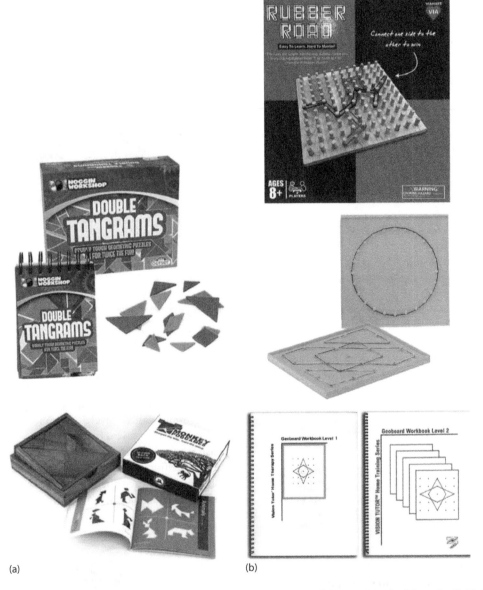

(a)   (b)

Figure 9.13 (a) Double tangrams. (b) Rubber Road. ([a]: Courtesy of Outset Media, Victoria, British Columbia, Canada; [b]: Courtesy of Mike Hart.)

Set-up

- Tangram pieces are placed before the patient and is shown the relationships between the edge lengths of each piece.

Procedure

1. Starting at the appropriate level, the patient is asked to fill the pattern with the blocks.
2. Begin with small groupings of pieces (i.e., 2, 3, 4) and move to 5 piece and 7 piece designs.
3. Commercially available patterns usually require all seven shapes and are, therefore, substantially harder.

Notes

- Some versions are wood construction and are less susceptible to jarring during use.
- Business card magnets can be attached and used in conjunction with a metal plate to further facilitate patients with tremors.
- This can be used for *visualization* if the clinician asks the patient to create the pattern with a left, right, vertical, or horizontal rotation (advanced).
- Unless specific pattern books are used, tangrams are performed off-pattern and are thus more difficult than other techniques.
- The clinician can make simple patterns that the patient will copy if standard designs are too complicated.
  - This is often an excellent start point when visualized transpositions will be used.

Availability

- Amazon.com and Outset Media

Geoboard/Rosner patterns (Figure 9.13b)

Purpose

- To develop the ability to perceive the position of objects in relation to oneself and other objects
- To be used as a tool for improving visualization
- To be used in an office or at home

Equipment

- Geoboard (usually 5 × 5)
- Rubber Board™ (VIAHART)
- Geoboard workbooks (Bernell)
- Rosner workbooks

Set-up

- For Geoboard and Rubber Board, the patient is given the pattern board, pattern to be copied, and a supply of rubber bands.
- For Rosner patterns, the patient is given the pattern printouts, blank pattern forms, and a pencil.

Procedure

1. Beginning with the appropriate level of difficulty, the patient is asked to make an exact copy of the template using either the rubber bands or pencil.
2. Self-detection of errors is to be encouraged especially if the procedures will be performed at home.

Notes

- The paper and pencil version of the technique is usually harder than the rubber bands.
- Geoboard workbook from Bernell.com comes with grease pen to make targets reusable.

Variations

- Given the proper grids, which can be made by the practitioner, geoboard shapes can be drawn rather than made with rubber bands similar to the Rosner technique.

Availability

- Amazon.com (boards and workbooks)
- Bernell.com (boards and workbooks)

Pentominoes™/Parquetry (Figures 9.14 through 9.16)

Purpose

- To develop the ability to perceive the position of objects in relation to oneself and other objects
- To be used as a tool for improving visualization
- To be used in an office or at home

Equipment

- Pentominoes
- Parquetry Blocks™
- Learning Resources Pattern Block Activity Pack™

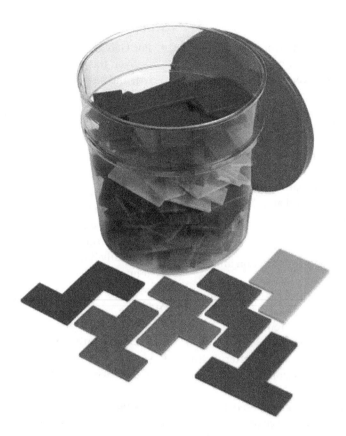

Figure 9.14 **(See color insert.)** Pentaminoes. (Courtesy of learningresources.com.)

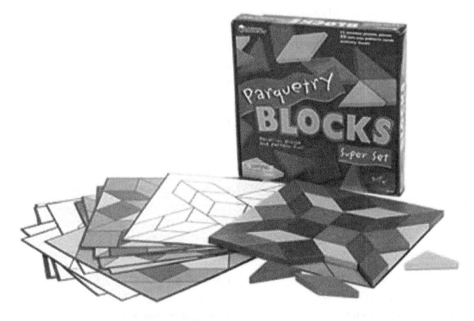

Figure 9.15 Parquetry Blocks. (Courtesy of learningresources.com.)

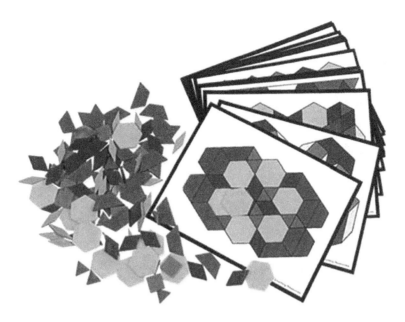

Figure 9.16 Parquetry Blocks. (Courtesy of learningresources.com.)

Set-up

- The patient is seated before a flat surface.
- Based on the patient's level of ability, the appropriate pattern card is chosen.

Procedure

1. The patient is given an appropriate pattern and asked to duplicate it.
2. The design should at first be constructed directly on top of the pattern card.

Notes

- As skills develop, the patient can be asked to make the figure off the pattern.

Variations

- To make for a simpler exercise, the patient can be asked to copy smaller patterns created by the clinician.
- This can be used to develop visualization skills by having the patient recreate the pattern rotated left, right, etc.

Availability

- Amazon.com

Pegboard activities (Figure 9.17)

Purpose

- To develop the ability to perceive the position of objects in relation to oneself and other objects
- To be used as a tool for improving visualization
- To be used in an office or at home

Equipment

- Any of the various peg and pegboard packages available
  - HABA Color Pegs™ (Amazon)
  - Pegboard techniques (Amazon)
  - Pegboard Activity Cards (www. teacherspayteachers.com)
  - More patterns available from many sources
- A series of cards is suggested but patterns can be created by the clinician:
  - Complex patterns can be too sophisticated for some patients.
- Lego pieces can be used for more 3D techniques
  - Standard size and large (Duplo™)

Set-up

- The patient is given pegs and a pegboard appropriate to the style of pegs used.

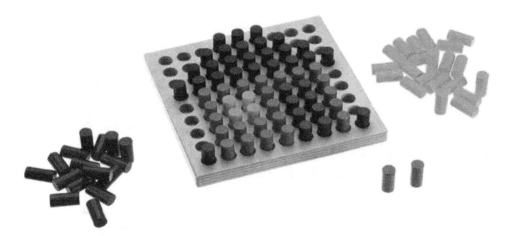

Figure 9.17 HABA Color Pegs. (Courtesy of HABA™, Skaneateles, NY.)

Procedure

1. The patient is instructed to match the given book or clinician pattern.
2. The patient is encouraged to perform the task visual rather than by counting pegs and spaces.

Notes

- Larger-size pegs and boards are available if the patients have a motor control problem.
- This can be used to develop visualization if the clinician asks the patient to create the pattern with a left, right, vertical, or horizontal rotation (advanced).
- Rather than use cards, simple patterns can be made by the clinician.

Availability

- Amazon.com (pegs, pegboards, patterns)
- www.teacherspayteachers.com (patterns)

Pegboard: CPT (Figures 9.18 and 9.19)

Purpose

- To develop the ability to perceive the position of objects in relation to oneself and other objects
- To be used as a tool for improving visualization

Equipment

- CPT computer program

Set-up

- The clinician sets the complexity of the pattern by selecting the appropriate "stimuli type" and starting screen.
- Direct copy is suggested for all starting out patients.

Procedure

1. The patient is told to copy the pattern in the left-side panel onto the one on the right.
2. The clinician should help the patient develop strategies to reinforce the learning process.
3. When the patient feels they have completed the pattern correctly, the word "DONE" is pressed and the correct answer is shown. If incorrect, the option is given to continue or retry.

Notes

- Although this technique can yield excellent results, many patients learn faster if they have real pegs in their hand and use a real pegboard.
- This available for home use in the PTS II system.

Variations

- As patients progress, the clinician can further go for basic visualization therapy by asking the patients to rotate their answer based on the options in the "stimulus mode."

Availability

- http://www.visiontherapysolutions.net

Additional home therapy techniques

Rush Hour

- See discussion in the section on visual sequential memory.

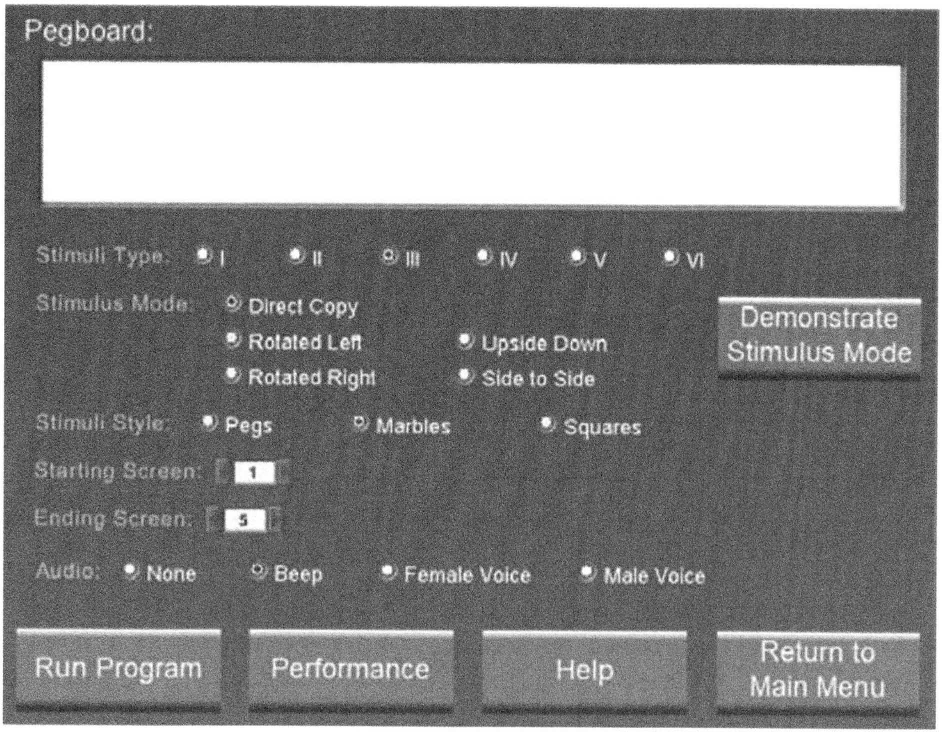

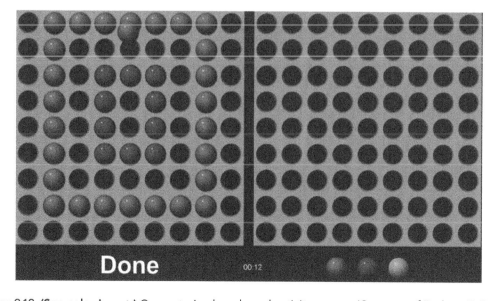

Figure 9.18 Computerized pegboard set-up screen. (Courtesy of Rodney K. Bortel.)

Figure 9.19 **(See color insert.)** Computerized pegboard activity screen. (Courtesy of Rodney K. Bortel.)

Visual discrimination workbook

- See discussion in the section on "Visual Discrimination."

Visual closure (Figures 9.20 and 9.21)

Purpose

- To develop those skills that enable a person to see an incomplete shape or object and, based on knowledge, logic, and experience, to infer the true nature of that object by mentally filling in the missing details. This is considered to be somewhat related to visual discrimination. It requires a degree of abstract reasoning.

Equipment

- CPT computer program

Set-up

- The patient is seated before the computer at an appropriate working distance (usually 16″–18″).
- The target type is determined; the degree of difficulty is variable and often related to the individual patient's needs and abilities. A good

start would be the use of letters though numbers would be easier.
- Rather than go with the default setting of 25 trials, it is better to have 3 runs of 10 trials.

Procedure

1. The patient is told he will see a "target letter" slowly being formed. He must determine from the four samples presented as follows the target which letter is a match.
2. The patient is told to find a point of balance between speed and accuracy.

Notes

- This is available for home use on the PTS II system.
- As is often the case, a wonderful home technique is jigsaw puzzles of the appropriate level of difficulty (described under visual discrimination).

Variations (both increase difficulty)

- With *sequential targets*, the possible answers are flashed one at a time. When the patient feels they can identify the answer, they press the space bar.

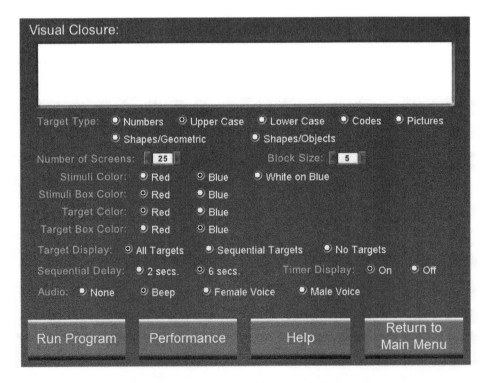

Figure 9.20 Visual closure set-up screen. (Courtesy of Rodney K. Bortel.)

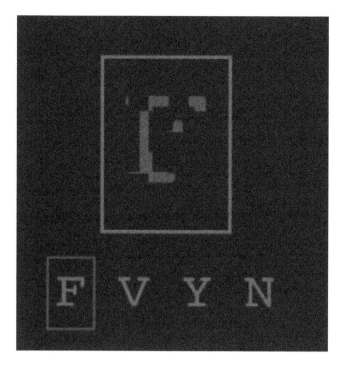

Figure 9.21 Visual closure activity screen. (Courtesy of Rodney K. Bortel.)

- A memory component can be added by selecting "no targets." When the patient feels they know the answer, they press the space bar, the target disappears, and they must choose from the four possible answers.

Availability

- http://www.visiontherapysolutions.net

Visual-motor integration (Figure 9.22)

Purpose

- To develop those skills that enable a person to see an incomplete shape or object and, based on knowledge, logic, and experience, to infer the true nature of that object by mentally filling in the missing details

Equipment

- Various commercially available dot-to-dot books based on the patient's abilities
- Harder examples
  - *1000 Dot-to-Dot* series (Thomas Pavitte—author) PR publicity

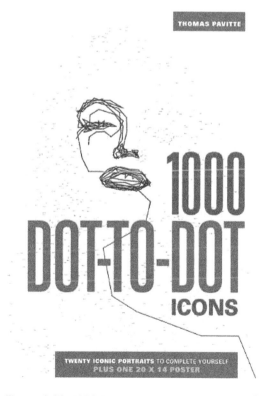

Figure 9.22 1000 Dot-to-Dot Icons. (Courtesy of Thunder Bay Press, San Diego, CA.)

- *The Greatest Dot-to-Dot Book in the World* (David Kalvitis—author) monkey around
- *Dots!: Super Connect-the-Dots Puzzles* (Conceptis Puzzles—author)

Set-up

- The following should be used: dot-to-dot patterns, pencil, and ruler (optional).

Procedure

1. The patient is asked to solve the dot puzzle in the conventional way but to pay careful attention to using visual cue to guess the ultimate identity of the target.

Notes

- This technique may also help to reinforce fine motor control.
- This is similar in concept to "creating line designs" but has a more advanced figure–ground demand.

Variations

- Use of a ruler may facilitate better success with the patients having motor control difficulties.

Availability

- Amazon.com (authors noted earlier)

Creating line design books (Figure 9.23)

Purpose

- To enhance the ability to coordinating visual perceptual skills together with gross and fine motor movement, that is, to integrate visual input with motor output
- To help improve bimanual motor control
- To be used in an office or at home

Equipment

- Skill appropriate line design book
- Pencil with eraser
- Ruler

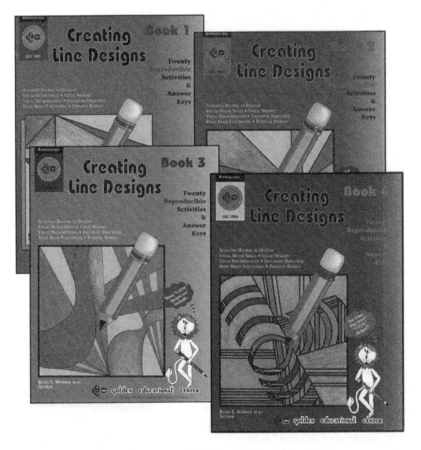

Figure 9.23 *Creating Line Designs*. (Courtesy of Golden Ed, Redding, CA.)

Set-up

- Materials are laid out on an appropriately large table with lighting appropriate to the patient's needs.

Procedure

1. The patient is told to read the instructions as to the proper sequence to make a shape (letters first vs. numbers first).
2. The patient then connects the numbers to the same numbers and letters to the same letters to reproduce the image exactly as seen in the sample.
3. The patient should be asked if their reproduction matches the target image. If not, ask the patient where the differences lay.

Notes

- This is similar in concept to Dot-to-Dot series but has a more advanced cognitive component.
- Four books available with increasing difficulty.

Availability

- www.rainbowresource.com
- http://www.goldened.com

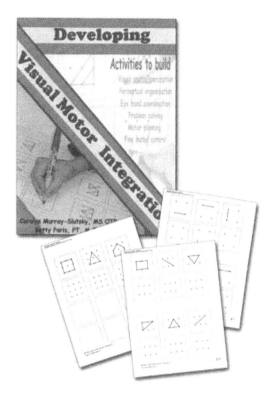

Figure 9.24 Developing Visual-Motor Integration.

Developing visual-motor integration (Figure 9.24)

Purpose

- To enhance the ability to coordinating visual perceptual skills together with gross and fine motor movement, that is, to integrate visual input with motor output
- To help improve motor control as needed
- To be used in an office or at home

Equipment

- One of the five available Developing Visual-Motor Integration books available based on the patient's level

Set-up

- The patient is given a pencil and the appropriate level design book.

Procedure

1. The clinician asks the patient to copy the design onto the grid beneath.
2. Generally, a ruler is not used (see "Notes" section below)
3. Erasures are not only permitted but encouraged so that the final product is a match of the original image.

Notes

- There are five levels based on the patient's ability.
- The levels are 4, 6, 9, 16, and 25 dots.
- A ruler can be used if motor skills are substantially reduced but this should be short term as the primary goal is to develop fine motor control. Use of a ruler will only develop the ability to make the visual match.

Variations

- Similar techniques
  - Rosner
  - Geoboard

Availability

- www.therapro.com

Visual tracing: CPT (Figures 9.25 AND 9.26)

Purpose

- To enhance the ability to coordinating visual perceptual skills together with gross and fine motor movement, that is, to integrate visual input with motor output
- To help improve bimanual motor control

Equipment

- CPT computer program

Set-up

- The clinician sets the number of lines, the start and end screens, and whether the patient will enter their response with the mouse or keyboard.

Procedure

1. Using the mouse, the patient is asked to track the cursor over the line from the specified letter to the appropriate number.
2. The patient is told that the computer will keep track of the time the procedure took, the percentage of time the patient is on the line, and whether the answer is correct.

Notes

- For VMI purposes, the use of the mouse should be the limiting (therapeutic) component. The number of line should be kept to a minimal level at the beginning.
- As the patient improves, more lines should be added. This will also increase difficulty by adding to the figure–ground demands of the exercise.
- For pure eye movement therapy, the mouse is actually supportive.
- The speed should not be emphasized early in this technique.

Availability

- http://www.visiontherapysolutions.net

Visual sequential memory (Figure 9.27)

Purpose

- To improve and develop the short- and long-term memory

Equipment

- CPT computer program

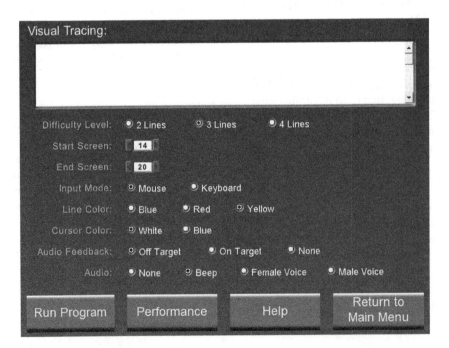

Figure 9.25 Visual tracing set-up screen. (Courtesy of Rodney K. Bortel.)

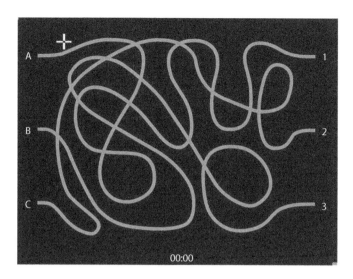

Figure 9.26 Visual tracing activity screen. (Courtesy of Rodney K. Bortel.)

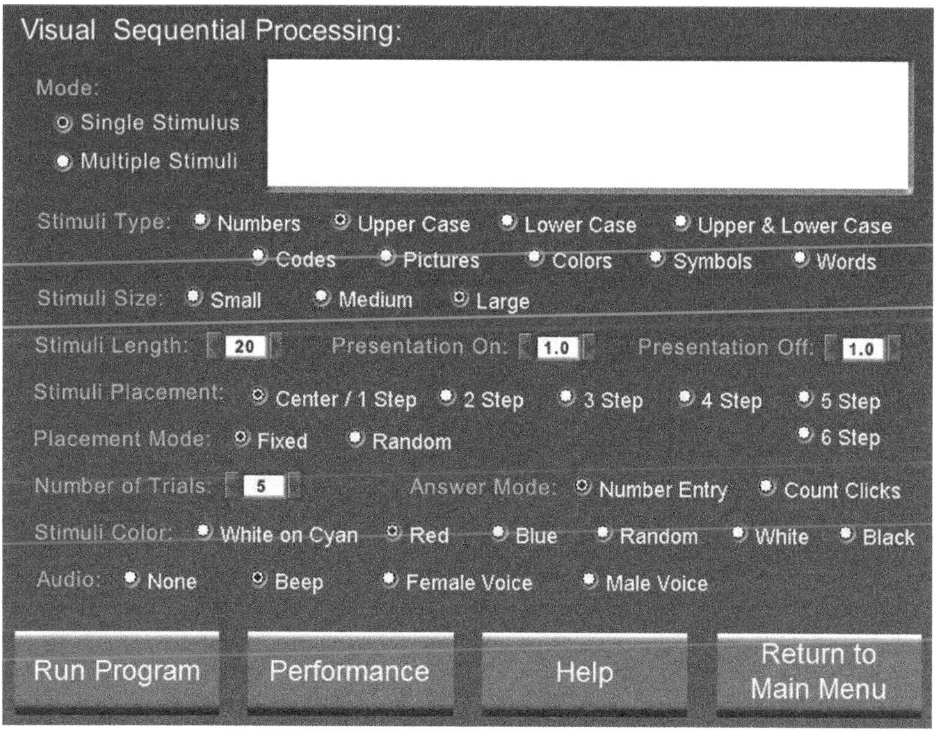

Figure 9.27 Visual sequential processing set-up screen. (Courtesy of Rodney K. Bortel.)

Set-up

- Provide many available options. It is best to begin with numbers as there are less options and distractors.
- It is also best to start with centrally placed stimuli.
- The stimuli length should be as long as the patient can tolerate.

Procedure

1. The patient is told they will be shown a number of characters. The first one they see is the target. They must keep track of the number of times the original target is seen and enter the total (number entry) or press the space bar each time the target is displayed (count clicks).

Notes

- Stimuli placement determines where the target will appear on the screen.
- Placement mode determines whether the target will stay in one place or vary.
- Stimuli length determines how many characters will be shown in a trial.
- Peripheral stimuli in conjunction with prisms can be good with patients having visual neglect.

- Difficulty can be increased by
  - Increasing the number of steps in stimuli placement
  - Using a random placement mode
  - Using pictures, colors, or symbols as the stimulus type
  - Increasing the stimuli length

Variations

- Available for home use with limited parameter adjustability on the PTS II system

Availability

- http://www.visiontherapysolutions.net

Visual span CPT/PTS II (Figure 9.28)

Purpose

- To improve and develop the short- and long-term memory

Equipment

- CPT computer program

Set-up

- Start with an appropriate level and option profile for the patient.

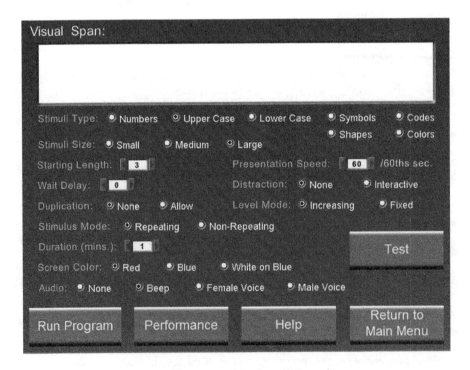

Figure 9.28 Visual span set-up screen. (Courtesy of Rodney K. Bortel.)

- Set the starting length, stimulus type, duration of trials, and mode (to repeating or nonrepeating).

- **Procedure**

1. The patient is told they will see a series of targets. At the end of the sequence, they will be asked to enter them into the computer in the same order they were displayed. With each correct answer, the sequence will lengthen by one element. If an error is made, the number of elements in the sequence will restart at the original length.

Notes

- Numbers are easier as there are less options.
- Repeating mode is easier as the sequence will get longer but not change.
- Fixed-level mode is the easiest as the length of the sequence does not increase.
- Be careful of the presentation speed. Too fast or too slow will make the task more difficult.
- To further increase difficulty:
  - Use symbols or shapes as they are harder to verbalize.

- Allow duplication (an element can appear more than once).
- Utilize a wait delay: The patient can only enter the answer after a brief time out.
- Use the distractor: The patient will have a simple task to perform before entering their response.

Variations

- Available for home use with limited parameter adjustability on the PTS II system

Availability

- http://www.visiontherapysolutions.net

Visual memory CPT (Figures 9.29 and 9.30)

Purpose

- To improve and develop short-term sequencing skills
- To be used to further develop short-term spatial memory skills

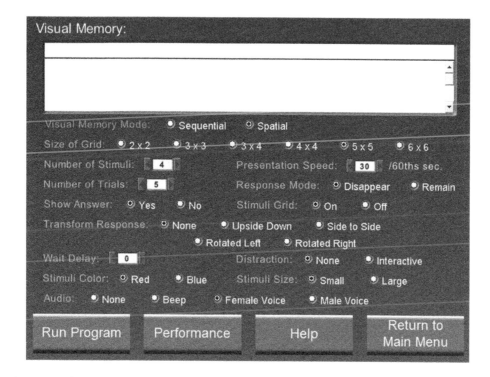

Figure 9.29 Visual memory set-up screen. (Courtesy of Rodney K. Bortel.)

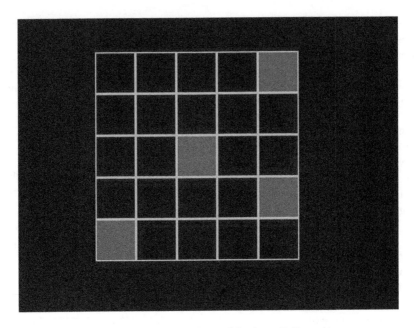

Figure 9.30 Visual memory activity screen. (Courtesy of Rodney K. Bortel.)

Equipment

- CPT computer program

Set-up

- It is best to begin the sequential component with a demonstration of the spatial memory mode.
- Make all settings to coincide with the patient's abilities.

Procedure

1. Set memory mode to special, size of grid to 3 × 3, number of stimuli to 3, and presentation speed to default.
2. Inform the patient that the computer will display three red squares for ½ second. They will then be asked to identify the previously marked squares with the mouse.
3. If this is successful, then use the same parameters (or decrease the number of stimuli to 2) and inform the patient the targets will light up in a sequence. They will then have to repeat the sequence with the mouse.

Notes

- When set to spatial mode, the sequencing task is removed and only location of the targets is of concern. This does not really make the task easier but different.

- Transform response: task can be made extremely difficult by asking the patient to rotate their answer left or right.
- Be careful of presentation speed. Too fast or too slow will make the task more difficult.

Variations

- Response mode: "disappear" briefly displays the patient answer while "remain" keeps it displayed.
- A distractor can be added that will demand the patient commits the sequence to memory for a longer period of time.

Availability

- http://www.visiontherapysolutions.net

Rush Hour (Figures 9.31 through 9.33)

Purpose

- To improve and develop the short- and long-term memory
- To further develop the cognitive concept of a rational sequence
- To improve visualization skills

Equipment

- Any of the commercially available Rush Hour series of games

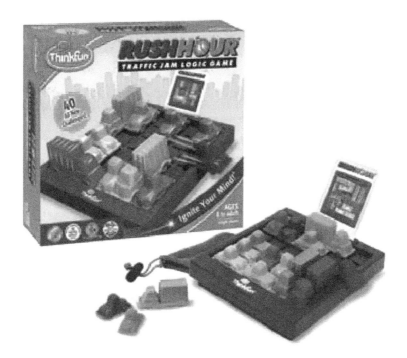

Figure 9.31 Rush Hour. (Courtesy of Thinkfun, Alexandria, VA.)

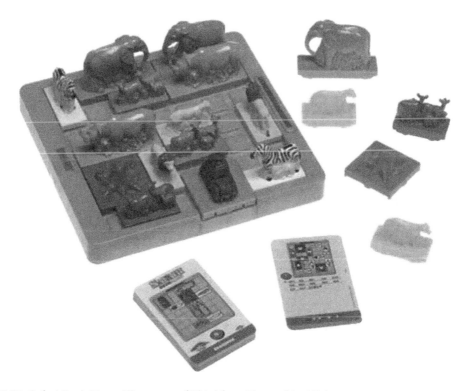

Figure 9.32 Safari Rush Hour. (Courtesy of Thinkfun, Alexandria, VA.)

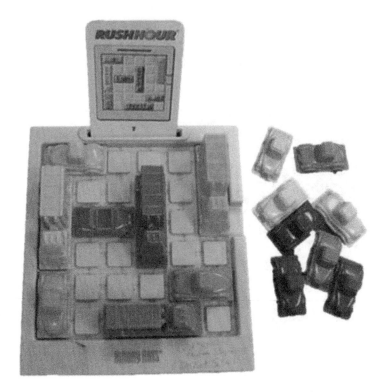

Figure 9.33 **(See color insert.)** Rush Hour. (Courtesy of Thinkfun, Alexandria, VA.)

Set-up

- Select a game style (see below) based on the patient's abilities.
- Select a card appropriate to the patient's abilities.

Procedure

1. The clinician instructs the patient to populate the playing surface with the exact components on the card.
2. The goal is to get the appropriate card off of the board while moving the pieces in only one direction.

Notes

- It is always a good idea to start with the simplest card to teach the technique.
- Rush Hour Jr. is simple as there are unit 1 × 2 unit pieces.
- Rush Hour standard is somewhat harder as there are both 1 × 2 and 1 × 3 unit pieces.
- Rush Hour Safari is the most challenging as the grid is larger and there are 1 × 2, 1 × 3, and 4 × 4 unit pieces.

Variations

- Although this is not true to the sequential memory goals of the exercise, for patients where the task is beyond their reach, the clinician can ask the patient to move the pieces in the answer sequence described on the reverse of each card to develop auditory visual processing skills.

Availability

- Thinkfun

Visual spatial memory (Figures 9.34 and 9.35)

Purpose

- To develop and improve spatial memory skills

Equipment

- CPT computer program

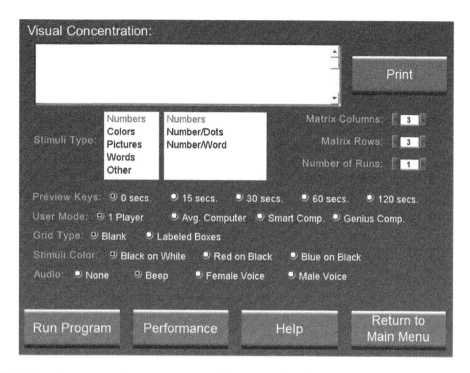

Figure 9.34 Visual concentration set-up screen. (Courtesy of Rodney K. Bortel.)

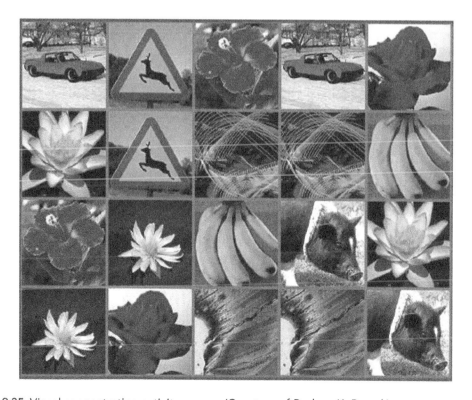

Figure 9.35 Visual concentration activity screen. (Courtesy of Rodney K. Bortel.)

Set-up

- Begin the program with the difficulty level appropriate to the patient's abilities.
- The best starting point is a 15 second preview and a 3 × 3 grid with numbers although some patients perform better with pictures.

Procedure

1. The patient is told they will see a series of targets for 15 seconds and they should remember the locations of the pairs and use the mouse to key in the matches.

Notes

- Difficulty can be increased by
  - Increasing the size of the grid
  - Changing targets to colors

Variations

- With the preview key set to zero there is no preexposure. The patient should be told to expose pairs of squares from left to right and top to bottom, only moving back when they see a target that would make a match to a newly exposed square.

Availability

- http://www.visiontherapysolutions.net

Improving Visual Memory, units 1 and 2 (Figure 9.36)

Purpose

- To develop and improve spatial memory skills

Equipment

- Book 1 or 2 based on the patient's abilities (a good idea to always start with book 1)

Set-up

- The patient is given an appropriate illuminated table and the page of the book to memorize.

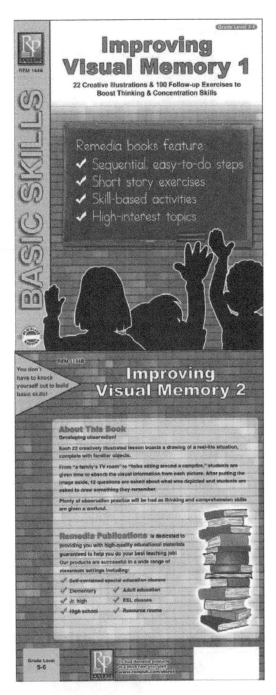

Figure 9.36 *Improving Visual Memory.* (Courtesy of Remedia publishing, Scottsdale, AZ.)

Procedure

1. The patient is given 2–3 minutes to remember as many of the objects in the picture (a complex line drawing).
2. After the time expires, the clinician asks the content questions on the following page.
3. If there are any missed answers, the clinician should give the patient 1–2 more minutes to look at the original picture and then the clinician repeats the missed questions.

Notes

- The patient should be encouraged to be aware of the spatial relationships to the objects in the picture.

Variations

- The patient could be asked to verbalize the picture as they study it to reinforce the visual memory.

Availability

- Remedia Publishing

Tic-tac-toe with memory component (Figure 9.37)

Purpose

- To improve spatial memory skills

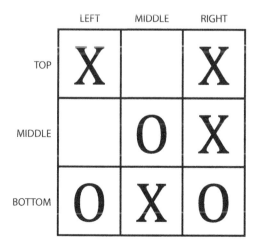

Figure 9.37 Tic-tac-toe with memory component.

Equipment

- Paper and pencil
- Premade tic-tac-toe grids that make the technique easier
- A clipboard to act as a visual mask

Set-up

- The patient is seated opposite the clinician.
- The clinician has the tic-tac-toe grid and a pencil.

Procedure

1. The clinician covers the grid with the clipboard and makes an "X" on the tic-tac-toe grid.
2. The grid is shown to the patient for 5 seconds (less or more based on the patient's ability).
3. The patient is then asked where he would like to move and responds by saying upper, middle, or lower row and left middle or right column: that is, place an "O" in the top left square.

Notes

- Not all patients will have the cognitive skills to perform this technique. It would be wise to see if they have the capacity to perform tic-tac-toe without the memory component first.
- The technique can be made harder by shortening the display time.

Variations

- This can be used to further visualization skills as related to directionality: that is, the patient must give their answer based on the visual perspective of the clinician facing opposite them.
- The range of difficulty is added by using a 4 × 4 grid.

Availability

- Created by the clinician

Parquetry pattern matching with memory time out (Figure 9.38)

Purpose

- To improve spatial memory skills

Equipment

- Parquetry blocks (preferred) of various shapes
- Tangrams or Pentominoes
- A clipboard to act as a visual mask

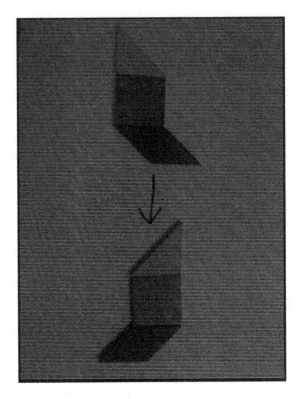

Figure 9.38 **(See color insert.)** Parquetry pattern matching.

Set-up

- The patient is seated across from the clinician
- The clinician arranges three to four Parquetry Blocks of different colors in a simple pattern protected from the patient's view by the clipboard.

Procedure

1. The patient is told they will briefly be shown a small grouping of blocks. They will then have to reproduce the pattern.

Notes

- This is similar to tic-tac-toe technique but stresses visual or verbal/cognitive.
- The patient should be helped to think of ways of visualizing the relationships of the different components of the group. This could include verbalization.
- It is best to start with square blocks as it will be easier to remember when the patient is asked to repeat the pattern.
- To make the task more difficult:
  - The triangles and/or parallelogram shapes can be added to the squares.
  - The duration of the exposure can be reduced.
  - The patient can be given larger patterns.
  - The patient can be given more shapes than needed to copy the pattern.
  - The patient can be asked to perform a transformation: left, right, side to side, or upside down.

Availability

- Amazon.com
- Optometric Extension Program Foundation (oepf.org)
- Bernell.com

SUNY Visual-Motor Forms (Figure 9.39)

Purpose

- To improve the speed of cognitive processing through repetition
- To be used to develop organization skills and bimanual integration
- To be used to develop laterality/directionality skills if necessary

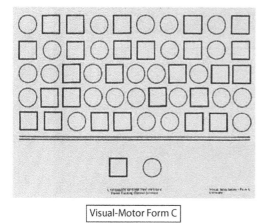

Visual-Motor Form C

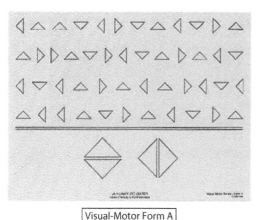

Visual-Motor Form A

Figure 9.39 Visual-Motor Forms C and A.

Equipment

- Appropriate visual-motor form based on the patient sophistication and needs

Set-up

- The patient is seated at a table with the appropriate visual-motor form.
- For form C: The patient is asked to place their left index finger on the lower square and the right on the lower circle.
- For form A: The patient is asked to place their left index finger on the up/down arrow group and the right on the left/right group.

Procedure

1. The patient is asked to move the appropriate finger to the top shape and then return to the "home" position: circle for circle and square for square on form "C" and the correct triangle on form "A."

Notes

- Do not start the technique with speed as the primary goal. Instead, develop organization and consistency first.
- To increase the difficulty, have the patient perform the exercise bimanually. Now the patient uses the targets as the "rule" for which of the "home" figures to touch.
  - Example for form A:
    - The patient pits their left finger on the "target" left pointing arrow and the right finger on the "home" left arrow.
    - Next, the patient pits their left finger on the *target* up pointing arrow and the right finger on the *home* up arrow.

Variations

- The patient can be asked to verbally name the shape as they land on the target and return *home*.
- This can be synchronized with a metronome.

Availability

- Online

Visual perceptual speed: CPT

This is performed exactly as described in the figure–ground section. Once the figure–ground component is mastered, the clinician should have the patient concentrate on developing speed. Stressing form recognition and peripheral awareness will accelerate the speed process.

Visual search: CPT/PTS II

As with perceptual speed, this technique is performed exactly as described in the figure–ground section. Once the figure–ground component is mastered, the clinician should have the patient concentrate on developing speed. Stressing form recognition and peripheral awareness will accelerate the speed process.

Perceptual speed: CPT (Figures 9.40 and 9.41)

Purpose

- To improve speed of cognitive processing through repetition

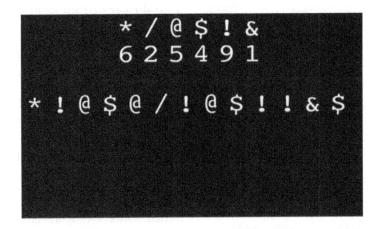

Visual Coding:

Response Type: ⊙ Numbers ● Letters ● Codes
Key Type: ⊙ Symbols ● Colors ● Pictures
Length of Key: [6]
Length of Stimulus: [20]
Number of Trials: [5]
Screen Color: ⊙ White on Black ● Red/Blue on Black
Audio: ● None ● Beep ⊙ Female Voice ● Male Voice

View Stimuli
Test Preview
Test

Run Program | Performance | Help | Return to Main Menu

Figure 9.40 Visual coding set-up screen. (Courtesy of Rodney K. Bortel.)

```
* / @ $ ! &
6 2 5 4 9 1

* ! @ $ @ / ! @ $ ! ! & $
```

Figure 9.41 Visual coding activity screen. (Courtesy of Rodney K. Bortel.)

Equipment

- CPT computer program

Set-up

- The patient is seated before the screen and an appropriate level of difficulty is entered into the settings.

Procedure

1. The patient is told that they will have to enter a specific response based on the key example on top of the screen:
   a. 6 for *, 2 for /, and 5 for @ in the following sample
      i. He will be assed for accuracy and speed of processing.

Notes

- As with other techniques, it is better to develop the skill untimed at first.
- Timing should begin as the skill is mastered.
- The technique can be made more difficult by lengthening the key sequence.

Availability

- http://www.visiontherapysolutions.net

Tachistoscope CPT/PTS II (Figures 9.42 AND 9.43)

Purpose

- To improve cognitive acquisition speed

Equipment

- CPT computer program

Set-up

- The patient is comfortably seated in front of the computer console.
- The parameters appropriate to the patient's abilities are entered.

- A good starting point would be three numbers at 30/60ths of a second with medium size.

Procedure

1. The patient is told the computer will quickly flash series of numbers after an auditory cue.
   a. The patient will then enter the numbers on the keyboard.
   b. As success is achieved, gradually decrease the presentation speed until it is tachistoscopic (0.1 second).
   c. Once a given level is manageable at 0.1 second (80% success would be a good goal), the next step is to add one element and start at the slower presentation speed of 30/60ths of a second.

Notes

- The technique is easier with numbers as there are less numbers (10) than letters (26) and they are in a predictable pattern on the keyboard.

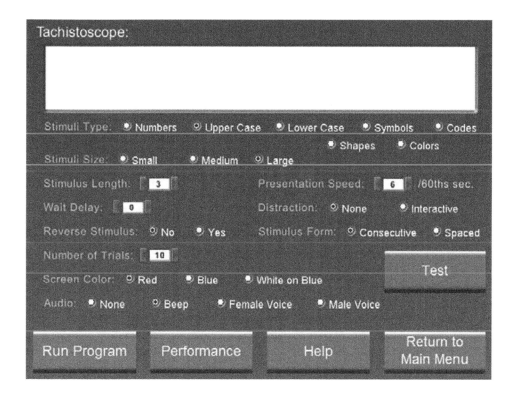

Figure 9.42 Tachistoscope set-up screen. (Courtesy of Rodney K. Bortel.)

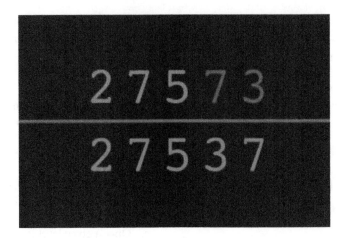

Figure 9.43 Tachistoscope activity screen. (Courtesy of Rodney K. Bortel.)

- The technique can be made more difficult with the delay parameter.
- This can be used at home as part of the PTS II program.
- Other tachistoscopic programs are available.

- In the aforementioned example, the red numbers were incorrect and the green were correct.

Availability

- http://www.visiontherapysolutions.net

10

Low-vision rehabilitation in TBI

INTRODUCTION

Low-vision rehabilitation is an excellent secondary source for management of patients with traumatic brain injury (TBI). Depending on the severity and effect from TBI, low-vision rehabilitation can be a great strategy for managing chronic and permanent secondary visual deficiencies. Although low vision is typically reserved for those with severe vision loss, the same tools a low-vision clinician uses can be applied to aid the functional vision of a patient suffering from TBI. In the majority of cases, patients suffering from TBI do not result in permanent or severe vision loss. However, severe injuries can cause permanent damage along the optic track, radiations, and the occipital lobe, which the visual information is interpreted. Damaging these essential visual pathways can result in low vision as well as other secondary TBI symptoms, ranging from accommodative spasms to homonymous hemianopia to complete cortical blindness. The clinician who is willing to treat and manage TBI must be prepared for strategies to deal with advanced cases of TBI. In this section, we will discuss the concepts and strategies to manage vision loss.

CONCEPTS OF MAGNIFICATION, FIELD ENHANCEMENT, AND CONTRAST SENSITIVITY

Magnification

Normal functional vision involves multiple different components for us to interpret color, depth, space, brightness, and movement (Campbell et al. 1970, De Valois and De Valois 1980, Hess 2011). We will discuss functional vision from a low-vision perspective with emphasis on its modifiable components: spatial frequency, contrast sensitivity, and visual field. Normal vision requires all three to be in good working order. We will first discuss the concept of spatial frequency and its relations with magnification.

Spatial frequency relating to vision is defined as the space between bands of light and dark (De Valois and De Valois 1980). The minimal amount of spacing a person can notice between the bands of light and dark is what we used to determine a person's visual acuity (Ginsburg 2003). This is often devised into the form of letters, shapes, or directionality to test an individual's ability to detect the minimal spacing difference between light and dark (Figure 10.1).

When damage occurs to the eye affecting visual acuity, the most effective way to improve spatial frequency recognition of the patient, such as reading speed and other functional tasks, is with magnification and low-vision aids (Virgili et al. 2013). This can also be applied to patients suffering from crowding affects as it effectively decreases the field of view and limits the amount of information the patient is able to see Leat et al. (1999) and Huurneman et al. (2013). There are roughly 8–10 different proposed methods to calculate how much magnification a patient may need when attempting to read (Cole 1993). The accuracy of those methods are variable, some studies suggest that using near acuity for calculating necessary magnification is more accurate (Thibos et al. 1996). However, no one method is effective 100% of the time. Thus, the easiest method may be most practical for determining a starting point during clinical examination. The simplest method is Kestenbaum's rule (Kestenbaum and Sturman 1956), which predicates that the add power necessary for the patient to read 1m acuity or 20/50 at near, is the inverse of the distance acuity.

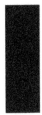

Two cycles, lower SF   Five cycles, higher SF

Figure 10.1 Representation of spatial frequency of two cycles versus five cycles.

Example 1:

If the patient's visual acuity is 20/100, the inverse would be 100/20 = 5. Kestenbaum's rule predicts that this patient can read 20/50 with +5.00D of add power.

Alternatively, one can use another simple method called the Sloan method. This is done with an M notation near card, either single letters or continuous text at 40 cm. The patient will read the lowest line possible with the best corrected Rx and +2.50 add. The additional dioptric power needed to achieve 1 m (20/50) near acuity is predicated by multiplying the patient's M notation acuity by 2.50.

Example 2:

The patient's near acuity is 3.2 m with +2.50 add. The total magnification needed to achieve 1.0 m acuity is 3.2 m × 2.5 = 8.00D. The patient will require an additional 8.00D of add to read 1.0 m acuity. Keep in mind the new closer working distance of 1/10.5D = 9.52 cm.

Although 1 m or 20/50 near acuity is newspaper size print, an important point to know is that providing the patient with magnification for threshold 20/50 near acuity is often not functional enough due to a variety of other factors such as contrast loss, metamorphopsia, and/or central/paracentral scotomas. Thus, the reading goal of the patient is the reading acuity the clinician should attempt to achieve and improve upon with magnification. If reading a normal print book is the patient's goal, usually 1 m print or 20/50 near acuity is the size we need to achieve. However, considering that the patient may have other deficiencies that will further decrease his functional ability, the reading acuity goal should be one to two lines smaller than 20/50 to give the patient some lead way for better function. An additional 30%–40% more dioptric power may be required to achieve the next line of near acuity. If patient is using +10.00 add, a total

of +13.00 or +14.00D will be needed to achieve the next line of acuity. This is due to the laws of linear magnification. As dioptric power increases and working distance decreases, each diopter becomes less effective in magnification. A good example would be the patient using a +10.00D added with a working distance of 10 cm. To increase 1x in linear magnification, we need to bring the working distance to 5 cm. This would equate to +20.00D! Changing the add power by 1 or 2 diopters in this case has minimal effect and should be avoided.

Non-low-vision practitioners often are afraid of using a high add power, considering a minimal increase in power is often adequate in achieving improvement in acuity for a normally sighted patient. This is not true for low-vision patients. Many beginner low-vision clinicians will try an additional +1.00 add repeatedly until they achieve the desired effect. In effort to avoid trial and error, additional chair time, and likelihood for patient frustration and fatigue, it is important to avoid trying arbitrary add powers to increase acuity. It is more efficient to follow a plan for magnification and adjust accordingly.

The same rule of magnification may be applied for TBI patients suffering from crowding effects; however, this is not a well-studied subject and can only be taken as theoretical and anecdotal evidence.

Contrast sensitivity

Contrast sensitivity is an essential part of vision that eye care professionals in optometry/ophthalmology seldom check. It is used in certain specialty practices in pediatric care and in low-vision evaluations; however, it is not always done with consistency or standardization. I do want to emphasize the importance of this matter as contrast loss can cause a severe functional deficit in vision. Without measuring or knowing the severity of loss, it is difficult clinically to predict the outcome of treatment or functional ability of the patient.

How do we define contrast sensitivity? It is simply the ability to tell between light and dark (Ginsburg 2003). Human contrast sensitivity works with spatial frequency for most functional tasks such as seeing a black pen on a black table or seeing the flight of stairs when descending. Without contrast sensitivity, we cannot appreciate spatial frequency (Figures 10.2 and 10.3).

This diagram shows the spectrum of visible versus invisible based on spatial frequency and

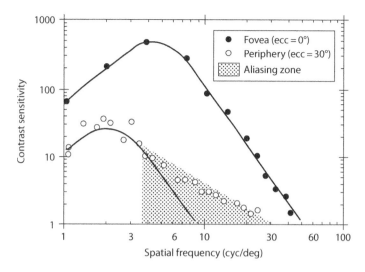

Figure 10.2 The line represents the threshold level of human visibility of an object with set contrast level and cycles of spatial frequency. Below the curve is visible, and above the curve is invisible. (Data from Thibos, L.N. et al., *Vision Res.*, 36(2), 249, 1996.)

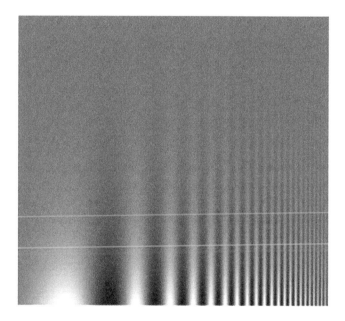

Figure 10.3 A visual representation of contrast sensitivity and spatial frequency from the visible spectrum to the invisible spectrum. (Data from Campbell, F.W. and Robson, J.G., *J. Physiol.*, 197(3), 551, 1968.)

contrast sensitivity. When contrast is reduced, lower spatial frequency is needed for target to be visible. This comes into play for our patients with damage to the eye as reduced acuity often come with reduced contrast.

How do we measure contrast sensitivity? There are many different ways to test contrast, most are based on a chart system involving letters, shapes, or spatial frequency. From anecdotal standpoint, I find contrast testing with letters the easiest as it usually comes in a smaller format with simple and fast testing protocols. Testing with spatial frequency gradient is somewhat unnatural and less practical to perform due to size, testing distance, and interpreting of data. Pelli–Robson chart has been extensively used for studies in contrast sensitivity and thus established itself as one of the gold standards of contrast testing (Elliott et al. 1990). The miniaturized version called the MARS test is essentially the same test giving at near instead of 1 m. According to Richman et al., MARS and Pelli–Robson contrast charts are the most reliable and easiest tests to administer (Richman et al. 2013).

Management of contrast sensitivity loss can be accomplished with magnification and colored filters when dealing with object or letter recognition. Filters that block blue light are the most effective in contrast enhancement as it blocks short-wavelength light and shows greater disparity between long and short wavelengths of light (Wolffsohn et al. 2000). If one is looking through a yellow lens, background or objects in the blue spectrum will appear darker, thus creating a greater difference in contrast. There is, however, an apparent subjective report of increased brightness with a yellow spectrum filter.

Often, patients with TBI respond negatively to increased stimulation; see previous sections regarding tints for reducing photophobia in TBI patients.

Field enhancement

TBI patients suffering from visual field loss are good candidates for visual field enhancement devices. Additional rehabilitation with an orientation and mobility specialist is part of this process. These patients will benefit the most from early referrals as they are having the greatest difficulties in the most acute phases of their condition. Visual field enhancement can be done in a variety of ways, depending on the type of field loss and the functional goal of the patient.

Hemianopic field loss

This type of field loss can be homonymous or nonhomonymous, meaning the field loss is either symmetrical or not. This depends on the location of damage along the optic radiations. The more occipital the damage, the more homonymous the field defect (Fadzli et al. 2013). Patients suffering from this condition often have functional defects with mobility, reading, and issues with activities of daily living (ADL) (Qiu et al. 2014). Damage to right cerebral hemisphere more so than left can result in neglect where the patient will completely ignore the contralateral side of visual field perceiving that it does not exist (Parton et al. 2004, Kim et al. 2008). Characteristic symptoms usually include missing half of their face when shaving, eating half their plate, etc. These patients also have severe functional difficulties getting from one place to another, typically bumping into obstacles on the side of their field loss. When reading, they will miss the beginning or the end of the sentence.

Management and functional improvement for patients with hemifield loss is a multifaceted approach as no one solution can completely solve all functional deficits. For mobility, the typical approach is with different types of prisms to shift images from missing field into seeing field (Smith et al. 1982, Woo and Mandelman 1983, Perez and Jose 2003). This can be achieved most economically with Fresnel prisms placed in half of spectacle correction from point of fixation toward missing field. Some sparring of the central field is preferred as to not affect patient's visual acuity (Figure 10.4). The power of the Fresnel also will need to be fairly high as 1-diopter prism is only equivalent to 0.59° of image shift.

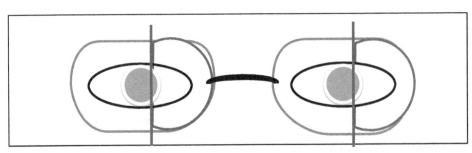

Figure 10.4 An example of Fresnel prism placement for a left homonymous hemianopic field defect with base-left prism. Avoid affecting the central vision by slightly displacing to the left of visual axis. The placement would be similar if the defect was on the right side.

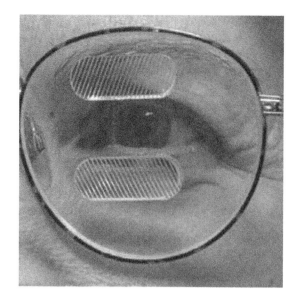

Figure 10.5 An example of proper placement of Peli prisms for left homonymous hemianopia. (Courtesy of Chadwick Optical Inc., Souderton, PA.)

The disadvantage is that the patient will have a large scotoma in visual field as head turning will be required to view into missing field.

Next option is the use of small sector prisms developed by Dr. Eli Peli (Brower et al. 2008, 2014) (see Figure 10.5). These have an advantage over the half lens prisms as it does not affect the direct horizontal field, thus no direct horizontal scotoma. These prisms are 40 PD or 57 PD strips placed above and below the eye on the side with visual field defect to give superior and inferior field enhancement. These come in several options of custom-made tape on strips or custom order with prisms ground into lens. These are more expensive if fabricated in lab; however, these can be fabricated in office with Fresnel tape on prisms.

A less popular option is the Gottlieb prism. These are circular high-powered prisms placed horizontally on one eye toward the side with field loss and provide image shift from the missing field for mobility purposes. The disadvantage of this system is the horizontal scotoma where the prism is located. It is, however, much smaller compared to full half prism placement as discussed previously.

Severe peripheral field loss

If there is severe traumatic brain damage resulting in 360° field loss, the patient will be much more challenging to rehabilitate. This type of damage can be cortical, orbital, or large bilateral cerebral involvement. Treatment approach typically requires multidispensary involvement from occupational therapy to adjust the patient for mobility and safety. These patients may also benefit from a guide dog once they have successfully mastered the use of the white cane.

From an optical standpoint, it is somewhat difficult to manage a patient with very little visual field such as 5°–10°. However, if the patient has larger useable field, a field enhancement system such as the channel prism design can be very beneficial if the patient can adept. These are high-powered prisms placed in each section of the lens around central field to shift image in from inferior nasal and temporal. The disadvantage is a large scotoma in all areas with prism; thus, the patient must turn head more to scan. Another method is to use a reverse telescope. This method may be accepted among the academic field, however, it is often clinically difficulty to accept, as the patient must sacrifice visual acuity to increase field. Very few of my patients have much success fitting and using reverse telescope systems.

Severe field loss patients will benefit most greatly from the use of a mobility cane and training with a mobility specialist. The mobility cane, white and red for legal blindness and yellow and white for visually impaired, are used much like a sonar with a sweeping motion to tell if there are any obstacles ahead. It is also helpful to maneuver up- and downstairs, as the cane can be used to judge the depth and distance of each staircase. If the patient masters the use of the cane, they can be eligible to apply for a guide dog, which is the next best thing to having sight again for some patients. These specially trained dogs can guide the patient safety across streets, avoid obstacles, and find entrances to buildings and other mobility assistance that are not possible with the cane.

Altitudinal field loss

Altitudinal field loss typically arises from damage at the level of the retina or optic nerve (Fraser et al. 2011). However, rare instances of altitudinal field defects can be a result of occipital lobe damage above or below the calcarine fissure (Holt and Anderson 1997, Luu et al. 2010). Depending on the superior or inferior nature of defect, different strategies are utilized for rehabilitation.

Superior field loss is less devastating for patients versus inferior field loss. Inferior field defects are associated with mobility difficulties, finding the next line when reading, finding objects on a table, and other ADL issues. Superior field loss is much more functionally adaptable as most of our functional tasks are not above our heads or significantly over our visual horizon. These patients may adapt well with some based down yoked prism. The amount of prism necessary may depend on the goal of the patient. If the inferior visual field is involved, base-up yoked prism may be used to aid the patient; however, the patient may require much more in-depth mobility training and use of cane to avoid obstacles.

LOW-VISION EXAMINATION WITH EMPHASIS ON TBI AND DEVICE SELECTION

Low-vision examination

Being trained as a medical professional, one can hear the phrase "history is everything" when it comes to examination, testing, and diagnosis of patients. We often base the examination and lab work or many of the components of a medical examination on the complaint of the patient and the history we get from them. Sometimes, the history alone provides enough detail to reach a diagnosis; examination then provides the findings to support the diagnosis. This is much the same in a low-vision examination; more importantly, history is required to identify a patient's functional deficits, safety concerns, and ultimate goal for rehabilitation.

When taking history on a low-vision exam, several major sections are generally involved. How are they functioning for viewing distance, viewing for near, ADL, and mobility? Some sample questions could be if the patient can identify street signs or signals to cross the street, or see people's faces. Can they see their mail or read the news headlines? Although more and more people are moving toward digital mediums where size and contrast are no longer issues, letters in the mail continue to be a problem for the modern-day low-vision patient.

The next biggest area is ADL functions at home, such as cooking, seeing the microwave, seeing numbers on a phone, and telling time. These are more essential as they threaten the patient's livelihood and may prompt immediate intervention.

Mobility is the next area of safety concern. Patients need to be assessed regarding their ability to get around safely, avoid bumping into objects, falling into ditches, tripping over obstacles, and seeing the stairs. Below is a list of function geared inquiry that can be used when taking a low-vision history:

Chief complaint: This is usually a patient complaining of difficulty in seeing and was being referred by another provider.

Ocular history: This includes diagnosis of condition, duration, treatments/surgeries, and follow-ups made by the doctor that is managing the condition.

Hobbies/goals: This includes the patient's goal for rehabilitation, e.g., watching TV, reading, and collecting stamps.

Functional ability questionnaire

Mobility (patients' ability to get around safely):
☐ Difficulty in seeing stairs and curbs
☐ Difficulty in seeing obstacles, dips, and potholes
☐ Difficulty in seeing street signs or signals
☐ Bumps into objects/people
☐ Recent history of falls

Activities of daily living (ADL):
☐ Difficulty in seeing numbers on a phone
☐ Difficulty in using microwave
☐ Difficulty in pouring liquids
☐ Difficulty in seeing to cook
☐ Difficulty in seeing food
☐ Difficulty in doing chores at home (laundry, cleaning, etc.)
☐ Difficulty in seeing colors
☐ Difficulty with price tags/product ID when shopping

Distance:
☐ Difficulty in watching TV (distance and screen size)
☐ Difficulty in identifying faces
☐ Difficulty in driving

Near:
☐ Difficulty in reading newspaper/mail
☐ Difficulty in reading handwriting
☐ Difficulty in reading headlines
☐ Difficulty in seeing computer
☐ Difficulty with small print

Lighting:
☐ Bothered by glare
☐ Sees better in bright lighting
☐ Sees better in dim lighting

With the completion of history, we then tailor the examination and device recommendation toward the goal they want to achieve. Most patients will have a goal to read better or see distance better. Some patients with recent vision loss may be in denial of their condition and believe that a pair of glasses will fix everything they have. These patients are often challenging and may not respond well to any advice or recommendation you give them. Do not be discouraged, as the patient go through the phases of acceptance, they will return for help. However, do demonstrate to the patient devices or aids that will allow the patient to perform at their goal; this will at least stick in their mind when they have accepted their condition.

The first component in the examination as with any type of eye examination is to check the patient's visual acuity. The preferred chart to use is the Early Treatment of Diabetic Retinopathy Study (ETDRS) chart. This chart is superior to all others over its flexible test distance, five letters for all acuity sizes, and variation of letter size based on logMAR values to give larger range of acuities compared to Snellen, which often miss letter sizes between 20/100 to 20/200 and 20/200 to 20/400. Many new electronic chart systems have incorporated this method; however, the screen size and test distance is often an issue. The ETDRS chart is tested in meters; original version is done at 4, 2, or 1 m. Newer editions have a 3 m test distance chart, equivalent to 10'. Conversion to Snellen is recorded with 10' over the letter size. When initially taking acuities, patients often need to be encouraged to perform the best they can. It is not their intention to malinger regarding their vision; however, they can potentially read two to three more lines by simply eccentric viewing and blur interpreting. It is essential to get the best possible baseline to avoid later confusion when refracting the patient, as they will often try extra hard to get more letters. Without a proper baseline, the examiner may be lead to believe they are making a bigger difference than they really are and ultimately prescribe an Rx based on this false assumption. This may result in a significant cost to the patient with little gain.

To achieve best results with refraction, it is often better to use a trial frame and loose lenses. Working inside a phoropter will limit the patient's ability to eccentrically view the chart, which can result in a less accurate finding; the phoropter can also trigger symptoms of post-traumatic stress disorder as it can evoke feels of claustrophobia in a TBI patient due to its unnatural and closed environment. When performing refraction, it is also important to demonstrate lens options between large values in a range of what is called just noticeable difference (JND). This concept is important because a patient with 20/200 vision will not appreciate the difference between 0.25D difference typically in a phoropter. The JND is made to calculate the amount of power necessary for a patient with X acuity to see a difference. This value can be calculated by using the denominator divided by 100. If a patient's vision is 20/400, the JND this patient can perceive is $400/100 = 4D$. By bracketing the patient with four diopter difference in lenses, in this case a +2D and a –2D, the patient should be able to tell if vision is better toward the plus or minus direction. Here are two simple methods to calculating what bracketing lens to use.

Method 1: Inverse of the patient's acuity divided by 10

Example:

1. The patient's acuity is 20/200. Its inverse value is $200/20 = 10$. Divide the value by $10 = 1$. Thus JND bracketing lenses $= \pm1.00D$. When refracting this patient, it is best to use a plus and minus 1.00D lens to fine-tune the Rx.
2. The acuity is 20/150.
   - Inverse: $150/20 = 7.5$
   - Divided by 10: $7.5/10 = 0.75$
   - Final bracketing lenses $= \pm0.75D$

Method 2: Denominator divided by 200

1. VA: 20/320
   a. $320/200 = 1.6D$ or $\pm1.60D$.
   b. No such lens is typically in trial frame set, so it is best to round up to $\pm1.75D$.
   c. When bracketing, always round up your lens power to the next closest lens. Rounding down is never a good idea due to the difference in power that may be below the patient's threshold.

Once refraction is completed and the best possible correction is determined, an assessment of functional vision needs to be completed before moving on to devices' recommendations. These functional tests are the ones we have discussed in Chapter 1, such as testing for scotoma in central field, peripheral field test, and contrast sensitivity test. These tests will determine additional functional deficits in addition to visual acuity, which will aid in device selection and recommendation.

Next step is to calculate the patient's predicated magnification needed based on acuity. We need to take into account the patients' additional deficits here as well; more power may be needed if severe contrast or paracentral scotomas/metamorphopsias are involved.

Near low-vision aids

The best optical aid for patients with only low-power needs is simply spectacles with the appropriate add power. Magnification at the spectacle plane provides the maximum field while maintaining two hands free for viewing of books, newspaper, or whatever the near target may be. This method works with linear magnification, which is explained with the analogy of looking at the New York skyline and being at the foot of the Empire State building. The object is magnified 1× if the distance is decreased by 1×. If patient is normally viewing objects at 40 cm, bringing object to 20 cm will provide 1× power in magnification. The limitation is the patient's comfort level. Other consideration is also binocularity. As working distance decreases, convergence demand increases. This is calculated with the formula PD (cm) × working distance (diopters) = convergence demand.

Example:

1. If patient is working at 40 cm and has a PD of 60 mm, the convergence demand is
   a. $6.0 \times 2.5D$ (1/0.4 m) = 15-diopter prism of convergence demand.
2. If same patient brought working distance to 10 cm, the new convergence demand is
   a. 6×10 (1/0.1 m) = 60-diopter prism.

Convergence is extremely uncomfortable and sometimes a physical impossibility for patients with high power. Base-in prism can be placed in Rx to alleviate convergence demand; however, high-powered prism will lead to chromatic aberration and degrade image quality. If spectacle high add is necessary, monocular is the preferred choice. These can be custom fabricated in lab or prefabricated options can be dispensed in office if no significant astigmatism is involved. These come in binocular with base-in prism already ground in or monocular types without prism. For high-powered monocular versions, the Clearimage II spectacle microscope made by Designs for Vision Inc. has high-quality optics with minimal edge distortion. Another system that can be utilized is the clip on add. This goes up to 7× in power (28D) and can be clipped on the spectacles. They allow for a 10 cm increase in working distance at the cost of field of view versus at the spectacle plane. It is an alternative if the patient is strongly against a close working distance. See Tables 10.1 and 10.2 for range of powers and appropriate working distances.

Table 10.1 Popular prefabricated spectacle microscopes with power and appropriate working distances

Prism half-eye/ full-eye readers	Several different manufacturers, styles, and designs available	Optelec (shoplowvision.com, Eschenbach, Coil, and others)
Dioptric power	Prismatic power	Working distance (cm)
+4.00	6 Δ BI each eye, total 12 Δ	25
+5.00	7 Δ BI each eye, total 14 Δ	20
+6.00	8 Δ BI each eye, total 16 Δ	17
+7.00 (less common)	9 Δ BI each eye, total 18 Δ	14.3
+8.00	10 Δ BI each eye, total 20 Δ	12.5
+10.00	12 Δ BI each eye, total 24 Δ	10
+12.00	14 Δ BI each eye, total 28 Δ	8.3
+14.00 (less common)	16 Δ BI each eye, total 32 Δ	7.1

Sources: Data obtained from Eschenbach optic, Eschenbach.com, July 26, 2015; Optelec US Inc., Shoplowvision.com, July 26, 2015.

Table 10.2 Spectacle microscopes from designs for Vision Inc. with power and appropriate working distance

Clearimage II monocular microscopes OD or OS, fellow lens is plano	Manufacturer, Designs for Vision Inc.	Working distance
Dioptric power	Magnification	(cm)
+8.00	2×	12.5
+12.00	3×	8.3
+16.00	4×	6.25
+20.00	5×	5
+24.00	6×	4.1
+28.00	7×	3.6
+32.00	8×	3.1

Source: Data obtained from Designs for Vision Inc., Designsforvision.com, August 1, 2015.

Handheld magnifiers and stand magnifiers

Magnification with magnifiers is another good option for patients with vision loss. The powers range from 8D to 56D, which covers most of the spectrum of vision loss. However, there is a significant problem with handheld magnifiers at higher powers. There can be significant edge distortion and can cause blur with minimal tilting or movement from focal point of lens. From the $8–10×$ (28–56D) range and up, it is often better to go to a stand magnifier system where the reading material has a set distance to be placed exactly underneath the stand mag. At this range of magnification, field of view is significantly reduced. Thus, for a more efficient view of the printed material, the stand magnifier lens should be placed as close to the eye as possible. Another important difference between handheld and stand magnifiers is what is needed at the spectacle plane. Handheld magnifiers if held at the focal point do not require accommodation, thus no add power is required. Stand magnifiers usually have a divergent wave front, typically requiring a small of add, no more than +2.50D. One final consideration when selecting magnifiers is the manufacturer, which label the powers differently. There are typically two

formulas for determining labeled magnification: F = diopters of magnifier and M = magnification, that is,

$$F/4 = M$$

or

$$F/4 + 1 = M$$

An 8D magnifier can be labeled 2× or 3× depending on the manufacturer; thus, it is very important to consider magnifiers in diopters and not the labeled magnification power (Tables 10.3 and 10.4).

If working distance needs to be maintained, another method of magnification is with spectacle-mounted telemicroscope. These are custom-made spectacles with the desired magnification in a telescopic system mounted in the lens at a position to view near targets with whatever working distance the patient desires. The magnification range is from 1.5× to 8× and there are various designs to suit different needs (Table 10.5).

ELECTRONIC DEVICES

Traditional electronic magnification for patients has been done on a closed-circuit television (CCTV). These devices have made little evolution since their debut and all have the basic magnifying of an image from camera to screen with a range of magnifications and color options. However, newer generations have been rapidly changing to keep up with more mainstream technology such as the iPad and other tablet formats. Most new CCTVs have optical character recognition (OCR) technology built in, which will read printed text to patient. The complexity and interface differs between models; however, they are essentially similar magnification devices with variable contrast settings. These devices are great for poor contrast sensitivity and poor visual acuity. Or if patient has severe photophobia, the reverse contrast on these devices can be less stimulating for the eyes.

Other devices to consider are the new tablet systems. These are intended for the mass consumer; however, certain models have been very user friendly and designed with accessibility in mind. The best example is the iPad by Apple, which offers great deal of features for its tablet and iPhone series. The notable features are reverse contrast, zoom, text to speech, and Siri. Reverse contrast completely inverts the color spectrum of color on the screen of the iPad and iPhone, making

Table 10.3 Handheld magnifiers from multiple manufacturers with range of powers and focal distance of specific powers

Dioptric power	Labeled magnification	Manufacturers, Optelec (O), Coil (C), Schweizer (S), Eschenbach (E), and other brands (*)	Working distance (material to magnifier) (cm)
8D	3×	O/C/S	12.5
9D	3×	O/C/S/E/*	11.1
10D	3.5×	O/S/E	10
12D	3× or 4×	Eschenbach, Optelec	8.3
16D	4× or 5×	O/C/S/E/*	6.25
20D	5× or 6×	O/C/S/E/*	5.0
24D	6× or 7×	O/C/S/E/*	4.1
28D	7× or 8×	O/C/S/E	3.6
32D	8× or 9×	C	3.1
38D	10×	E	2.6
39D	9.75 or 10.75×	O/S	2.6
40D	11×	C	2.5
48D	12× or 13×	O/S	2.1
50D	12.5×	E	2.0
56D	14× or 15×	O/S	1.8

Sources: Data obtained from Optelec US Inc., Shoplowvision.com, July 26, 2015; Eschenbach optic, Eschenbach.com, July 26, 2015; Coil CTP Inc., Coil.co.uk, July, 26, 2015.
Note: * Indicates other smaller brands not listed in the table.

Table 10.4 Stand magnifiers from multiple manufacturers with range of powers

Dioptric power	Labeled magnification	Manufacturers, Optelec (O), Coil (C), Schweizer (S), Eschenbach (E), and other brands(*)
8D	3×	O/C/S
9D	3×	O/C/S/E/*
10D	3.5×	O/S/E
12D	3× or 4×	Eschenbach, Optelec
16D	4× or 5×	O/C/S/E/*
20D	5× or 6×	O/C/S/E/*
24D	6× or 7×	O/C/S/E/*
28D	7× or 8×	O/C/S/E
32D	8× or 9×	C
38D	10×	E
39D	9.75 or 10.75×	O/S
40D	11×	C
48D	12× or 13×	O/S
50D	12.5×	E
56D	14× or 15×	O/S

Sources: Data obtained from Optelec US Inc., Shoplowvision.com, July 26, 2015; Eschenbach optic, Eschenbach.com, July 26, 2015; Coil CTP Inc., Coil.co.uk, July, 26, 2015.
Note: * Indicates other smaller brands not listed in the table.

Table 10.5 Spectacle-mounted telescopic systems from multiple manufacturers with range of powers and field of view and if near adaptations can be used

Manufacturer	Device	Magnification	Field of view	Range of focus
Eschenbach	MaxDetail	2×	20°	±3.0D
Eschenbach	Spectacle-mounted monocular or binocular wide field 2× telescope	2× (varies depending on reading cap)	22°	Reading cap +3D to +12D
Eschenbach	Spectacle-mounted monocular or binocular 2.5× telescope	2.5× (varies depending on reading cap)	13°	+3D to +16D reading cap
Beecher	Mirage head-mounted binocular or monocular telescope	3.4×, 4×, 4.5×, 5.5×, 6×, 7×, 8×	15° to 8°	+0.5 to +8D cap
Ocutech	Sightscope (spectacle mounted)	1.7× 2.2×	26° 18°	Infinity to desired near distance with custom reading cap
Ocutech	VES Sport (spectacle mounted)	4× 6×	12.5° 9.6°	23 cm to infinity; 30 cm to infinity; can use near cap
Ocutech	VES mini (spectacle mounted)	3×	15°	23 cm to infinity; cannot use cap
Designs for Vision Inc.	Full diameter (spectacle mounted)	1.4×, 1.7×, 2.2×, 3×, 4×	28° to 6°	Infinity to desired near distance with custom reading cap
Designs for Vision Inc.	Politzer bioptic design or full diameter design (spectacle mounted)	1.7×, 2.2×, 3×	28° to 8°	Infinity to desired near distance with custom reading cap

Sources: Data obtained from Eschenbach optic, Eschenbach.com, July 26, 2015; Ocutech Inc., Ocutech.com, August 1, 2015; Designs for Vision Inc., Designsforvision.com, August 1, 2015.

the background dark versus the bright letters. This makes patients with photosensitivity much more comfortable when reading with this setting. Zoom is another good feature built into the iPad/iPhone operating system. It allows zooming of any screen such as the menu or in app screens that normally do not respond to pinch zooming. On browser or text where regular zooming is already at maximum, the zoom feature will allow further zoom, which is helpful for anyone with severe acuity loss. If, however, there is little to no usable vision, the next step is to use the text to speech feature, which would speak everything that is on the screen. With Siri integration, patients that have little to no usable vision can dictate to the iPhone or iPad commands, questions, and other phone/tablet functions, and it will be performed without having the need to search for them. Additional use of camera with zoom and high contrast can simulate CCTV-like functionality. This makes the iPad/iPhone more versatile than any other operating format such as Windows- or Android-based systems. Android and Windows are not completely without accessibility features. Both have built-in features; however, they are not as intuitive and newer versions have mostly imitated methods Apple has used in their OS. Android is an open-source software and free for any manufacturer to use and modify. Most manufacturers do not invest the additional time to add software for accessibility-friendly use. The standard features are talkback, which reads text on screen, and Explore by Touch, which reads what is under the finger. Additional features include changing font size and some magnification. Windows smartphone/tablet devices have similar features to Apple with high contrast,

Table 10.6 Accessible Apple iPhone/iPad, Android, and Windows apps and software

System	Function	Cost
iPhone apps		
ZoomReader	OCR	$19.99
LookTel Money Reader	Reads bills from 20 countries	$9.99
Color ID	Recognizes colors	Free
VizWiz	Recognizes objects via software or human volunteer	Free
TapTapSee	Recognizes object	Subscription
NFB-Newsline	Provides news and magazines in text and speech options	Free app, needs subscription to service
Android apps		
Eyes Free Project*	Open-source apps to making Android devices accessible	Free
Windows Programs		
ZoomText	Magnifies screen and cursor, enhances contras, and also provides text to speech	$599
JAWS	Allows for interaction with PC based on audio feedback and keyboard commands	$895
CDesk	20 core programs for most PC functions with simple interface and PEGGY speech recognition	$595

Sources: Data obtained from Apple Inc., iTunes, July 25, 2015a; Apple Inc., Apple.com, July 26, 2015b; Google Inc., Eyes Free Project, August 1, 2015; Ai Squared, ZoomText, August 1, 2015; Freedom Scientific Inc., JAWS, July 26, 2015; AdaptiveVoice LLC, CDesk, August 1, 2015.

Note: * Indicates other smaller brands not listed in the table.

narration, and zoom with different gesture methods. The following are some apps that can be used (Table 10.6).

For some patients with severe vision loss, there are a few gadgets that are helpful for ADL. Many of these devices have ultimately been reimagined in the form of a smartphone app. For example, the Colorino by Care Tec, which identifies colors of objects, or the i.d. mate Quest® barcode reader can help low-vision patient identify items in a store by scanning the barcode. A new frontier that is underway is the spectacle-mounted camera systems that maybe a new way people with vision impairment can become much more functional. Their functions vary from OCR to face recognition, recognizing street signals, objects (brand symbols, common everyday objects), bus numbers, watching TV, etc. The complexity of devices ranges from simple camera and magnification system to built-in computer system with AI-like user interface capable of learning to improve its function

and use for users. Also under development is the new self-driving car technology, which will eventually enable our patients to be more independent.

TEAM APPROACH TO MANAGING TBI PATIENTS AND THEIR REHABILITATION

Optometrists have been established as the primary eye care physicians and a gateway for patients to seek further specialized care. Patients who suffer from TBI especially fit into this category. Their traumatic events may have damaging effects on any number of cerebral functions. A thorough evaluation from a neurologist is needed to rule out other deficits and referred to the appropriate rehabilitation specialist. As an optometrist, we can rehabilitate their binocular, accommodative, and visual processing systems with therapy and optical aids; however, there is much more than any one profession can cover. Appropriate referral to a low-vision specialist should be done to help with visual field loss, significant decrease in vision acuity, or contrast. Occupational therapy may be needed to help managing visual field loss, mobility, and management of safety and ADL at home. A physical therapist may be needed to help the patient with stability, coordination, muscle strengthening, and perhaps the use of a support cane. Patient may also need a speech pathologist, a psychologist, and a social worker to successfully rehabilitate and reenter into society. An essential component of our evaluation is to realize the additional needs a patient may have and help facilitate the referral process, so our patients start sooner on the road to recovery.

REFERENCES

Brower, A.R., Keeney, K., and Peli, E. 2008. Community-based trial of a peripheral prism visual field expansion device for hemianopia. *Archiv Ophthalmol.* 126(5):657–664.

Brower, A.R., Keeney, K., and Peli, E. 2014. Randomized crossover clinical trial of real and sham peripheral prism glasses for hemianopia. *J Am Med Assoc Ophthalmol.* 132(2):214–222.

Campbell, F.W., Nachmias, J., and Jukes, J. 1970. Spatial-frequency discrimination in human vision. *J Opt Soc Am.* 60:555–559.

Campbell, F.W. and Robson, J.G. 1968. Application of Fourier analysis to the visibility of gratings. *J Physiol.* 197(3):551–566.

Cole, R.G. 1993. Predicting the low vision reading add. *J Am Optom Assoc.* 64(1):19–27.

Combined Optical Industries Ltd. (COIL) www.coil.co.uk. July 26, 2015.

De Valois, R.L. and De Valois, K.K. 1980. Spatial vision. *Annu Rev Psychol.* 31:309–341.

Elliott, D.B., Sanderson, K., and Conkey, A. 1990. The reliability of the Pelli-Robson contrast sensitivity chart. *Ophthalmic Physiol Opt.* 10(1):21–24.

Fadzli, F., Ramli, N., and Ramli, N.M. 2013. MRI of optic tract lesions: Review and correlation with visual field defects. *Clin Radiol.* 68(10):538–551.

Fraser, J.A., Newman, N.J., and Biousse, V. 2011. Disorders of the optic tract, radiation, and occipital lobe. *Handb Clin Neurol.* 102:205–221.

Freedom Scientific Inc. JAWS. July 26, 2015.

Ginsburg, A.P. 2003. Contrast sensitivity and functional vision. *Int Ophthalmol Clin.* 43(2):5–15.

Google Inc. Eyes Free Project. August 1, 2015.

Hess, R.F. 2011. Early processing of spatial form. In: P.L. Kaufman, A. Alm, L.A. Levin, S.F.E. Nilsson, J. Ver Hoeve, and S. Wu, eds., *Adler's Physiology of the Eye*, 11th edn., pp. 613–626. Amsterdam, the Netherlands: Elsevier.

Holt, L.J. and Anderson, S. 1997. Bilateral occipital lobe stroke with inferior altitudinal defects. *Optometry* 71(11):690–702.

Huurneman, B., Boonstra, F.N., Verezen, C.A., Cillessen, A.H.N., van Rens, G., and Cox, R.F.A. 2013. Crowded task performance in visually impaired children: Magnifier versus large print. *Graefes Archiv Clin Exp Ophthalmol.* 251:1813–1819.

Kestenbaum, A. and Sturman, R.M. 1956. Reading glasses for patients with very poor vision. *Arch Ophthalmol.* 56: 451–470.

Kim, E.J., Choi, K.D., Han, M.K., Lee, B.H., Seo, S.W., Moon, S.Y., Heilman, K.M., and Na, D.L. 2008. Hemispatial neglect in cerebellar stroke. *J Neurol Sci.* 275(1–2):133–138.

Leat, S.J., Li, W., and Epp, K. 1999. Crowding in central and eccentric vision: The effects of contour interaction and attention. *Invest Ophthalmol Vis Sci.* 40:2504–2512.

Luu, S.T., Lee, A.W., and Chen, C.S. 2010. Bilateral occipital lobe infarction with altitudinal field loss following radiofrequency cardiac catheter ablation. *BMC Cardiovasc Disord.* 10:14.

Parton, A., Malhotra, P., and Husain, M. 2004. Hemispatial neglect. *J Neurol Neurosurg Psychiatry.* 75(1):13–21.

Perez, A.M. and Jose, R.T. 2003. The use of Fresnel and ophthalmic prisms with persons with hemianopic visual field loss. *J Vis Impair Blind.* 97:173–176.

Qiu, M., Wang, S.Y., Singh, K., and Lin, S.C. 2014. Association between visual field defects and quality of life in the United States. *Ophthalmology* 121(3):733–740.

Richman, J., Spaeth, G.L., and Wirostko, B. 2013. Contrast sensitivity basics and a critique of currently available tests. *J Cataract Refract Surg.* 39(7):1100–1106.

Smith, J.L., Weiner, I.G., and Lucero, A.J. 1982. Hemianopic Fresnel prisms. *J Clin Neuroophthalmol.* 2:19–22.

Thibos, L.N., Still, D.L., and Bradley, A. 1996. Characterization of spatial aliasing and contrast sensitivity in peripheral vision. *Vision Res.* 36(2):249–258.

Virgili, G., Acosta, R., Grover, L.L., Bentley, S.A., and Giacomelli, G. 2013. Reading aids for adults with low vision. *Cochrane Database Syst Rev.* 23:10.

Wolffsohn, J.S., Cochrane, A.L., Khoo, H., Yoshimitsu, Y., and Wu, S. 2000. Contrast is enhanced by yellow lenses because of selective reduction of short-wavelength light. *Optom Vis Sci.* 77(2):73–81.

Woo, G.C. and Mandelman, T. 1983. Fresnel prism therapy for right hemianopia. *Am J Optom Physiol Opt.* 60:739–743.

Companies providing software and devices

Adaptive Voice LLC, CDesk. www.adaptivevoice.com. August 1, 2015

Ai Squared. Zoom Text. www.aisquared.com. August 1, 2015.

Apple Inc. iTunes. www.apple.com/itunes/. July 25, 2015a.

Apple Inc. www.apple.com. July 26, 2015b.

Designs for Vision Inc. www.designsforvision.com. August 1, 2015.

Eschenbach optik. www.eschenbach.com/. July 26, 2015.

Freedom Scientific Inc. JAWS. www.freedom scientific.com/Products/Blindness/JAWS. July 26, 2015.

Google Inc. Eyes Free Project. https://play.google.com/store/apps/developer?id=Eyes-Free+Project&hl=en. August 1, 2015.

Ocutech Inc. www.ocutech.com. August 1, 2015.

Optelec US Inc. www.shoplowvision.com/. July 26, 2015.

11

Psychology and mild TBI patients

Patients may present to brain injury specialists with persistent neurological symptoms months to years after the injury. While it may be easy to assume that the symptoms are directly caused by injury to the brain, one must consider the role of psychology in persistent postconcussion symptoms. In the past, the effects of TBI were poorly understood and many patients who suffered from brain injury–related cognitive, balance, and visual changes were undiagnosed and had to live their lives struggling to understand why they were having these symptoms. In the recent years, there has been a greater understanding of the mechanism of brain injury and how patients can have lasting symptoms due to neurological injury. This has been great, and specialties such as speech and language pathology, neurooptometry, and vestibular therapy have been invaluable in retraining the brain to overcome persistent deficits. Unfortunately, on the flip side, there has been a significant amount of overassociation of brain injury with cognitive, neurological, and physical symptoms (Broshek et al. 2015, 228). Many in the rehabilitation community are overlooking the premorbid and comorbid conditions that complicate the postconcussive patient. To put this into perspective, most patients recover within 3 months to 1 year from their mild TBI (Cassidy et al. 2014, S132). This should lead to the question, "What is keeping the rest from recovering?"

Next, I will list the most common causes (Broshek et al. 2015, 228):

1. Depression
2. Anxiety
3. Sleep dysfunction
4. Balance/dizziness deficits
5. Visual deficits
6. Cognitive deficits
7. Headaches
8. Pending litigation

The patient may have only one or many of these factors. This is where a multidisciplinary team approach is of great importance. With evaluations from many specialties whose expertise are in these areas, they are able to identify with more certainty the cause of the concussed patient's persistent symptoms.

Psychological disturbances can manifest in several ways for patients with mild TBI, such as emotional distress, anxiety, depression, and irritability. There are many patients who report an exacerbation of long-standing mild anxiety or depression after their TBI. For most patients, these issues are adequately addressed with psychological or psychiatric treatment and does not affect our treatment of their visual dysfunction. In cases where the clinical picture does not match the patient's reported complaints or level of impairment, there is often one of the following: psychological illness, other disease process, or malingering. It is not recommended to treat the patient based on symptoms alone; it is important to also carefully review their neurooptometric evaluation to develop a clinical picture, as postconcussive symptoms are not specifically to concussion; these same symptoms are found in healthy adults, chronic pain patients, and spinal injury patients, just to name a few (Broshek et al. 2015, 228). There is a recent study published in the *Journal of Brain Injury* that postconcussive symptoms were found present to a similar extent in participants with no head injury (34%) compared to those with mTBI (31%) (Dean et al. 2012, p. 14).

This study again pointed out that postconcussive symptoms are not specific to mTBI. Finally, treating a patient based on their symptoms and not on objective evidence of dysfunction is harmful to the patient. This raises the risk of iatrogenic disorder, that is, making the patient think they are worse than they are by validating unsubstantiated complaints with extensive treatments. The patients oftentimes become fixated on their somatic symptoms, where perhaps the main source of the symptoms is psychological.

TREATMENT FOR PATIENTS WITH PSYCHOLOGICAL COMORBIDITY

The first step in treating patients who are suspected to have significant psychological factors confounding their symptoms is to refer them to a psychologist or psychiatrist. The next step is to treat these patients conservatively. Addressing symptoms of photosensitivity and blurry vision with tinted lenses and correcting refractive error often does help in anecdotally. It is important to avoid darkly tinted lenses and discourage patients from wearing sunglasses indoors as this can cause the patient to be more light sensitive in the long term. Neurovision rehabilitation should be brief, functional, and goal oriented. There should be functional goals in place such as increasing tolerance for reading or driving.

TREATMENT PLAN

Reiterating the aforementioned points, the number of therapy sessions should be clearly defined and consists of four to six sessions with the aim of improving their functional visual symptoms.

This is a sample of a treatment plan:

1. Energy management
2. Palming
3. Tips for computer and electronic use
4. Photophobia compensatory strategies
5. Line guide
6. Colored overlays
7. Oculomotor—completion of the following exercises:
   a. Spoon pursuits
   b. Post-it saccades
   c. Hart chart
   d. Michigan tracking

REFERENCES

Broshek, D.K., De Marco, A.P., and Freeman J.R. 2015. A review of post-concussion syndrome and psychological factors associated with concussion. *Brain Inj.* 29:228–237.

Cassidy, J.D., Cancelliere, C., Carroll, L.J., Cote, P. et al. 2014. Systematic review of self-reported prognosis in adults after mild traumatic brain injury: Results of the international collaboration on mild traumatic brain injury prognosis. *Arch Phys Med Rehabil.* 95(3):S132–S151.

Dean, P.J., O'Neill, D., Sterr, A. 2012. Postconcussion syndrome: Prevalence after mild traumatic brain injury in comparison with a sample without head injury. *Brain Inj.* 26(1):14–26.

Appendix: Templates/Extras

To be given to the patient by the front desk:

Post-trauma Vision Survey

Please rate the following symptoms on a scale of 0–4 (where 4 = severe).	
Visual history	
Blurry vision at distance	
Blurry vision at near	
Difficulty in transitioning between distance and near	
Pressure or pain behind or around eyes	
Covering/closing one eye to see more clearly	
Double vision	
Fatigue/eyes feeling tired when reading or looking at the computer	
Headaches when reading/performing visual tasks	
Losing your place when reading	
Dizziness	
Loss of balance	
Difficulty in busy visual environments, i.e., mall/supermarket	
Restricted field of vision/reduced peripheral vision	
Sensitivity to light	
Difficulty with nighttime driving	
Burning, itching, redness, or tearing of eyes	
Other visual symptoms not listed	

Traumatic Brain Injury Initial Visual Evaluation

Patient name: Age: Date:	
Appt time:	
Chief complaint: The patient is here for evaluation of vision and sensory motor function following	
Date(s) of incident:	
Other History of TBI	
Visual history	Initial
Blurry vision at distance	—
Blurry vision at near	—
Difficulty in transitioning between distance and near	—
Pressure or pain behind or around eyes	—
Covering/closing one eye to see more clearly	—
Double vision	—
Fatigue/eyes feeling tired when reading or looking at the computer	—
Headaches when reading/performing visual tasks	—
Losing your place when reading	—
Dizziness	—
Loss of balance	—
Difficulty in busy visual environments, i.e., mall/supermarket	—
Restricted field of vision/reduced peripheral vision	—
Sensitivity to light	—
Difficulty with nighttime driving	—
Burning, itching, redness, or tearing of eyes	—
Other visual symptoms not listed	

Ocular history	Medical history
LEE =	Diabetes =
LDFE =	HTN =
Eye injury/surgery =	Health problems =
Eye disease =	Medications =
Eye medications =	Medical allergies =
Flashes =	Family medical history =
Floaters =	

AutoR

AutoR			
OD		–	×
OS		–	×
PD			
AutoK			
OD			
OS			

Additional Entrance Testing

Color vision Ishihara OD /14 OS /14
Stereopsis: RDS, 250″; Wirt circles, 20″
NCT at by OD mmHg OS mmHg
VFE: OD: Reliability   Interpretation
OS: Reliability   Interpretation

Entrance Testing

HRx OD – × ADD
OS – ×
DVA OD 20/ OS 20/
NVA OD 20/ OS 20/
Pupils
EOM =
CVF OD OS

Sensorimotor Evaluation

Distance free space
DCT/VG =
DBI = / /
DBO = / /
Vertical =
Fixation dot = head shake =
W4D =

Near free space
Fixation Q =
Pursuits Q =
Saccades Q =
NCT/VG =
NBI = / /
NBO = / /
NPC = 2nd time =
NPC red lens =
W4D 16″ =

Refraction

Refraction
Retinoscopy OD = – ×
OS = – ×
Manifest OD = – ×
OS = – ×
BCVA   OD 20/20 OS 20/20 OU 20/20

Accommodation

Accommodation
FCC OD OS
NRA
PRA
(–) Lens amp OD OS
Near add OD OS
BCVA (near) OD 20/20 OS 20/20

Auxiliary testing
Vergence facility: BI — BO —
Tint trial: —
Banqueter foil occlusion
Occlusion density: —
Location: —
15-diopter yoked prism walk
Base-right response: —
Base-up response: —
Base-left response: —
Base-down response: —

Neuro Optometric Vision Rehabilitation

Session   of
DOE: —   Appt time: —
Diagnosis: 1.   2.   3.
Evaluation CPT 92012
Subjective
Demographics
Patient name: Age:
Chief complaint: The patient is here for vision rehabilitation of sensory motor deficits following
Date(s) of incident: Other history of TBI:
Current visual symptoms reported: 1.   2.   3.   4.   5.   Updated history: :   No changes in medical history   Ocular pain: Learning preference: Barriers to learning: Eval: Eval: :   Eval: :   Demo: Continue: *Therapy: CPT 92065*   1. Worked: 2. Worked: 3. Worked: 4. Worked: 5. Worked: Next: 1. Work: 2. Work: 3. Work: 4. Work:

Index

Printed and bound by CPI Group (UK) Ltd, Croydon, CR0 4YY

23/10/2024

01777692-0013